# Trauma Impacts

# Trauma Impacts

## The Repercussions of Individual and Collective Trauma

*Edited by*

Jessica Stone
Robert J. Grant
and
Clair Mellenthin

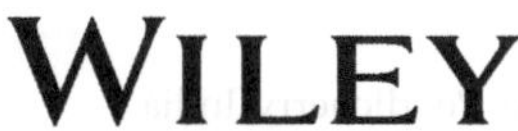

## SECTION III
## FUTURE IMPLICATIONS AND PROGRESSIVE SUPPORTS
## OF TRAUMA IMPACTS

# About the Authors

**Rachel A. Altvater, PsyD, RPT-S™**, is an award-winning, pioneering expert, leader, researcher, international trainer, author, and supervisor in the field of play therapy. She is a licensed psychologist in Maryland, Washington, DC, and Virginia, and she holds national certifications as a Registered Play Therapist–Supervisor™ and Certified Clinical Trauma Professional. She is the owner of Creative Psychological Health Services, co-owner of North Star Creations, past president of the Maryland/DC Association for Play Therapy, editorial advisory board member for the International Journal of Play Therapy®, and clinical consultant for Hopscotch. Dr. Altvater authored the book *Perspective: Contemplating the Complexities of Our Realities*, published her research in the *International Journal of Play Therapy* on technology use in play therapy, and is a contributing author in numerous scholarly texts.

**Liliana Baylon, LMFT-S, RPT-S**, is a bilingual and bicultural therapist fluent in Spanish and English. She holds a master's degree in counseling and marriage, family, and child therapy, and an MBA from the University of Phoenix. Specializing in treating trauma and multicultural issues in children and families, Liliana employs various therapeutic modalities, drawing on her expertise as a trained educator. Her therapy and supervision are enriched by her unique cultural perspective, fostering curiosity and inspiration. Passionate about professional development, Liliana offers workshops in mental health and cultural opportunities for diverse mental health and educational professionals, available in both English and Spanish.

**Steven L. Bistricky, PhD**, serves as the Associate Director of Clinical Training for clinical psychology programs at the University of Colorado Colorado Springs, directing the PhD trauma program and MA program. He is also an affiliate of the Lyda Hill Institute for Human Resilience. His research, teaching, and clinical supervision focus on adversity, trauma, adaptation, health, and growth with mindfulness and acceptance frameworks, concepts, and practices. His collaborative research, which often focuses on people's responses to disasters and interpersonal violence, has been published in leading academic journals.

**Isabella Cassina** is the Director of Project Management at the International Academy for Play Therapy (INA) based in Switzerland, Editor of *APTI's Play Therapy Magazine*, and Founding Member of the International Consortium of Play Therapy Associations. She is a social worker, registered therapeutic play specialist, PhD candidate in expressive arts therapy. Isabella is an author and expert in international cooperation and project development with over 10 years of international field experience in contexts of crisis and high vulnerability.

**Lisa Dion, LPC, RPT-S**, is an international teacher, creator of Synergetic Play Therapy, founder and president of the Synergetic Play Therapy Institute, co-founder of the Synergetic Education Institute, creator of the Business of Therapy, and host of the Lessons from the Playroom podcast. She is the author of Aggression in Play Therapy: A Neurobiological Approach for Integrating Intensity and is the 2015 recipient of the Association for Play Therapy's Professional Education and Training Award of Excellence.

**Jennifer Nelson Faulconer** is a nationally certified school psychologist with an Educational Specialist degree. Jen has over 15 years of experience working in schools. She focused on ameliorating the negative impacts of exposure to trauma or chronic stress, system-wide changes toward compassionate and effective discipline practices, positive behavior supports, and integrated service delivery. As students from racial/minority and low socioeconomic backgrounds often experience trauma disproportionately, Jen believes that trauma-informed care in schools is also a social justice issue. As a Colorado native, she enjoys spending active time outdoors with her family and dog.

**Jackie Flynn, EdS, LMHC-S, RPT-S**, a leader in trauma therapy, is known for her expertise in integrating play therapy, EMDR, and Gottman Method Couples Therapy. She is an advanced trainer for EMDRIA and an approved credit provider for the Association for Play Therapy. Jackie hosts global events like the Innovative Child Therapy Symposium and co-hosts the Playful EMDR Summit and Neuroscience of Play Therapy Summit. Her engaging presentations on nervous system-informed therapy, based on Dr. Stephen Porges' Polyvagal Theory, teach therapists worldwide. She offers mentorship and supervision, empowering therapists to integrate EMDR and play therapy. Jackie fosters a global play therapy community dedicated to transformative healing.

**Theresa Fraser** wears many hats. She has been a treatment foster parent for 30 years, an adoptive parent, a trauma specialist, an author, and is a Play Therapy

Supervisor. She is the owner of Maritime Play Therapy Centre in Nova Scotia/ Canada and Changing Steps Child and Family Counselling in Ontario and PEI Canada. She was the 2009 winner of the North American Trauma Award – Clinician of the Year, with the National Institute for Trauma and Loss . She was appreciative of having the opportunity to contribute to this valuable trauma resource with her beloved colleague Paris Goodyear Brown.

**Patricia Carolyn Gilbaugh** is a licensed independent social worker, Registered Play Therapist-Supervisor, certified mental health and nutrition specialist, and certified autism specialist at her private non-profit practice, Grace C Mae Advocate Center, located in Iowa. Patricia completed her doctorate and master's degrees in social work at the University of Iowa. Patricia specializes in working with medically complex and neurodivergent individuals and works with individuals of all ages. She also specializes in treating veterans with PTSD and providing family therapy for those with complex trauma. She has recently completed her certification in using food as medication for treating mental health conditions.

**Paris Goodyear-Brown, MSSW, LCSW, RPT-S**, and Approved EMDR Consultant, is the creator of TraumaPlay™, the Executive Director of the TraumaPlay Institute, the Clinical Director of Nurture House, and an Adjunct Instructor of Psychiatric Mental Health at Vanderbilt University. She is a Ted Talk speaker, a master clinician, and an internationally renowned presenter. She is a thought leader in the fields of child trauma and play therapy globally, received the APT award for Play Therapy Promotion and Education, served as the Executive Director of the Lipscomb Play Therapy and Expressive Arts Center., serves on the board of TNAPT, and has authored over twenty chapters and twelve books, including *Trauma and Play Therapy, Parents as Partners in Child Therapy,* and *Big Behaviors in Small Containers.*

**Robert Jason Grant, EdD, RPT-S**, is the creator of AutPlay® Therapy. He is a therapist, supervisor, and consultant and utilizes several years of advanced training and his own lived neurodivergent experience to provide affirming services to children and their families. He is an international trainer and keynote presenter and multi-published author of several articles and books. He is currently serving on the board of directors for the Association for Play Therapy.

**Fiona Hill, LPC,** is a licensed professional counselor-supervisor in Missouri and holds a national credential as a Registered Play Therapist™. She has extensive experience providing clinical services in nonprofit, government agency, and private practice settings. She is the owner of Lighthouse Play Therapy and Consulting Services, offering specialized therapeutic services in the areas of childhood trauma and attachment disruption, as well as supporting families impacted by varying developmental needs within the family system.

**Johnnie L. Jenkins, III, PhD,** is a licensed professional counselor, registered play therapist supervisor, and certified professional clinical supervisor. He taught at Argosy University. Dr. Jenkins was a counselor at the Morehouse School of Medicine. Dr. Jenkins's practice, the Jenkins Center, uses CBT and play therapy to treat families. Dr. Jenkins lectures on play therapy and legislative advocacy. Dr. Jenkins conducts training for the National Counselor Examination. He holds membership in several associations. His degrees include a Bachelor of Science in Biology from Mercer University, a Master of Arts Degree in Psychology from the Georgia School of Professional Psychology, and a Master of Philosophy and PhD in Public Policy from Walden University.

**Zara Kenigsberg** is a clinical psychology doctoral student with a focus on trauma psychology at the University of Colorado, Colorado Springs (UCCS). Zara received her BA in psychology, with a minor in biology, from Vanderbilt University. She now serves as the lab coordinator for the Cognition, Emotion, and Well-Being lab under the direction of Steven Bistricky, PhD. Her research focuses on the cognitive and emotional processes surrounding trauma disclosure, and she hopes to develop educational resources for the public about supporting trauma survivors.

**Betty S. Lai** is an associate professor at Boston College. Lai's research focuses on the impacts of the climate crisis and disasters on children. Her work has examined children's mental and physical health following large-scale disasters. Her work also examines how advanced statistical modeling strategies may be applied to better understand how to minimize the effects of disasters on children's functioning. Lai is dedicated to training the next generation of scholars. Lai's book, *The Grant Writing Guide: A Road Map for Scholars* (Princeton University Press), includes strategies and insights gleaned from her interviews with scores of grant writing experts.

**Julia Linger, MA,** is a doctoral student in clinical and school psychology at James Madison University. She is interested in promoting resilience and post-traumatic growth among children and families who have experienced trauma. Julia cares deeply about creating safe spaces in the therapy room and in communities, and she believes in the healing power of relationships.

**Clair Mellenthin, LCSW, RPT-S,** is a renowned clinical supervisor, international speaker, and acclaimed play therapist. As the author of best-selling book

Attachment Centered Play Therapy, she brings unparalleled expertise to the field. With a wealth of experience as a play therapist and professor, Clair has significantly impacted the lives of numerous children and families. Recognized for her contributions, she is a sought-after expert in media, frequently sharing insights on children and family issues at both local and national levels. Clair's commitment to advancing the understanding and practice of play therapy has positioned her as an influential figure, shaping contemporary therapeutic approaches for children and leaving an enduring mark on the field.

**Claudio Mochi** is the Director of the University Master's Program in Play Therapy of the International Academy for Play Therapy (INA) and the founder and president of the Association for Play Therapy Italy (APTI). He is a psychologist and psychotherapist, a Registered Play Therapist Supervisor™, an expert in emergency interventions and disaster mental health with over 20 years of international field experience. Claudio has presented on play therapy and trauma on 6 continents totaling over 20 countries and many more cities. He has authored books, chapters, and numerous articles.

**Mauricio Montes** is a counseling psychology doctoral student at Boston College and a National Science Foundation Graduate Research Fellow and Bill Anderson Fund Fellow. Mauricio's clinical work and research center on applying intersectional approaches to better understand trauma exposure, symptomatology, and recovery. Mauricio is dedicated to contributing to the improvement of the accessibility, inclusivity, and effectiveness of treatments for trauma and stressor-related disorders to foster affirming and empowering healing journeys.

**Hannah Jarrett** holds an Educational Specialist degree in Clinical Mental Health Counseling. She has experience working in public schools, rural integrated behavioral health, and community outpatient settings. She is a clinician at Secure Child & Virginia Attachment Center, where she provides attachment and trauma-informed therapeutic support to children and families and assists with evaluations of caregiver–child relationships. Hannah is committed to supporting the emotional and relational health of children with trauma histories and advocating for system-level changes to support children and families who are disproportionately exposed to chronic stress, marginalization, and violence.

**Alexa Riobueno-Naylor, MA,** is a counseling psychology doctoral student at Boston College and Bill Anderson Fund Fellow. Her research explores the intersection of multiple disaster exposures and mental health outcomes for youth. Riobueno-Naylor's clinical work focuses on serving youth and families using evidence-based, culturally informed interventions. She is dedicated to translating research findings into actionable insights that inform the development of effective prevention and intervention strategies for young people and their families.

**Margaret Ann Pauuw, PhD**, is an assistant professor at Eastern Michigan University and a licensed clinical social worker. Dr. Pauuw has been practicing social work since 2012, working mainly with people experiencing homelessness/housing insecurity and serious mental illness. Dr. Pauuw's research background includes social work practice in libraries and multidisciplinary treatment for youth and adults with psychosis.

**Mary Anne Peabody, EdD, LCSW, RPT-S**, is an associate professor at the University of Southern Maine, a licensed clinical social worker, a Registered Play Therapist Supervisor, and a retired K-12 school counselor. She has been a past board director of the Association of Play Therapy and received the 2019 APT Distinguished Service Award. Currently, she serves as Chair of the APT Foundation Board and on the editorial board of the International Journal of Play Therapy. A prolific author on play pedagogy in higher education and play therapy supervision, she presents internationally on a variety of topics, including feedback in play therapy supervision and the methodology of Seriously Therapeutic Play with LEGO®.

**Brian Quinones, EdD, LPC, ACS**, is a licensed professional counselor and a Registered Play Therapist Supervisor with a doctorate in Counseling Psychology. He is the co-owner of Gaming Approaches Towards Education, LLC in Edison, NJ. He uses an integrative gameplay approach to help individuals, families, and groups during therapy. Dr. Quinones uses gameplay to aid in developing healthier thoughts, feelings, and behaviors in our daily lives.

**Leanne Rohrbach-Stange, MSW, CSW**, is a Hematology Social Worker and Health Equity Specialist at Intermountain Health Primary Children's Hospital in Salt Lake City, Utah. Her areas of interest include working with children and their caregivers affected by acute and chronic illnesses who experience forms of grief associated with medical trauma. She takes great joy in playing outside, cuddling with kitties, dancing to live music, and traveling near and far with her husband.

**Jonathan B. Singer, PhD, LCSW**, is an internationally recognized expert in youth suicide and social work technology. He is Professor of Social Work at Loyola University Chicago, Past-President of the American Association of Suicidology, coauthor of two editions of the best-selling text *Suicide in Schools: A Practitioner's Guide to Multi-level Prevention, Assessment, Intervention, and*

*Postvention*, co-lead of the Social Work Grand Challenge "Harness Technology for Social Good," and founder and host of the award-winning Social Work Podcast, for which he was named a 2023 NASW Social Work Pioneer. He has chaired national committees for NASW and CSWE and served on advisory boards for Sandy Hook Promise, JED Foundation, Suicide Prevention Resource Center, and the 988 Suicide & Crisis Lifeline. He is the author of over 90 publications, and his research has been featured in national and international media outlets like *NPR, BBC, Fox, Time Magazine*, and *The Guardian*. In 2024, he was inducted as a Fellow of the Society for Social Work and Research. He lives in Evanston, IL, with his wife and three children and can be found on X/Twitter at @socworkpodcast and on Facebook at facebook.com/swpodcast.

**Shelby Somers, LSW**, is a licensed social worker (LSW) working towards clinical licensure in the mental health field. She received her master's in social work from Rutgers University and is a self-described "geek." Professionally, she has experience working with children, teens, and adults through traditional talk therapy and EEG Neurofeedback. Shelby is an LGBTQ+ and neurodivergent affirming therapist with experience working with individuals and families across the lifespan. She has previously presented on topics such as fandoms and identity, as well as trauma-informed tabletop role-playing. She is also interested in utilizing tabletop role-playing games and board games in a therapeutic setting.

**Anne Stewart, PhD, RPT-S**, is a licensed clinical psychologist and playful practitioner of therapy across the lifespan. Dr. Stewart's areas of teaching and scholarship include attachment and trauma-informed care, play therapy, couple and family therapy, crisis intervention, humanitarian demining/international stabilization, clinical supervision, interprofessional collaboration, and integrated behavioral health. With colleagues, she is an editor for *Play Therapy: A Comprehensive Guide to Theory and Practice*. She served as Chair of the Association for Play Therapy (APT) Board of Directors and founded the Virginia Association for Play Therapy. She is the recipient of the APT "Distinguished Service" Award, the Virginia Counselors Association's Humanitarian and Caring Person Award, the Virginia Outstanding Faculty Award, and was elected to the National Academies of Practice in Psychology.

**Jessica Stone, PhD, RPT-S**, is a licensed psychologist working in a private practice setting. She has been a practitioner, professor, presenter, mentor, and author for more than 30 years. Dr. Stone's interest in therapeutic digital tools, specifically using virtual reality, tablets, and consoles, has culminated in clinical mental health use and research for mental health, medical, and crisis settings. She is the co-creator of the Virtual Sandtray App for iPad (VSA) and the Virtual Sandtray for Virtual Reality (VSA-VR). Dr. Stone is the past Chief Psychology

Officer for AscendantVR, is a member of various boards, and serves as an affiliate of the East Carolina University College of Education Neurocognition Science Laboratory.

**Jose Tapia (he/him/his), PhD, CRC, LPC, RPT, NCC**, is an assistant professor in the Department of Counseling and Human Services in the College of Education at the University of Colorado Colorado Springs. He completed his PhD in counseling at the University of North Texas. Dr. Tapia's research agenda centers around disability-responsive practices in counseling across the lifespan. He is a Certified Rehabilitation Counselor, Licensed Professional Counselor, Registered Play Therapist, and National Certified Counselor. His clinical experiences have focused on serving clients with disabilities across the lifespan in English, Spanish, and American Sign Language. Finally, he has presented at the national, regional, state, and local level on topics related to graduate student success and mentorship, disability-responsive practices for serving people with disabilities, and bilingual counseling and supervision.

**Rachel Wethers** is a licensed clinical social worker in the states of Illinois, Michigan, and Missouri. She provides virtual therapy, specializing in trauma, attachment, anxiety, and neurodivergent needs and abilities. Rachel loves to be home with her fur family and friends or search the antique malls and garage sales for old-school games, toys, and memorabilia. www.thehopecheststl.com.

**David P. Yells** is a professor of Psychology at Texas A&M University-Texarkana where he teaches abnormal psychology, personality theory, and psychopharmacology. He earned a PhD in developmental psychobiology at the University of Nebraska before spending 18 years at Utah Valley University. His research interests include psychopathology, with a specific interest in substance use disorders. Together, David and Kris have 7 children and 13 grandchildren. They enjoy traveling, reading, and listening to a wide range of music.

**Kristine J. Doty-Yells, PhD, LCSW**, is a therapist and the Founding Director of the MSW program at Texas A&M University-Texarkana. She earned her MSW at Brigham Young University and her PhD from the University of Utah. Her practice experience includes individual and group therapy in a trauma clinic, at a residential educational center for adults with learning disabilities, and crisis counseling in an emergency room. Kris is also a popular presenter for social work trainings around cultural issues and ethics. In addition to her academic work, Kris maintains a small private practice.

# Prologue: Trauma Impacts

JACKIE FLYNN

What does it even mean to be human? In a consultation group with trauma therapists, a few years prior to this writing, I asked consultees to write down "To be human is ___________." 10 times on a sheet of paper. Afterward, I directed them to finish the sentences with words or phrases that quickly came to mind. It was astonishing to witness the variety of reactions. Some struggled with finishing the first sentence, while others completed the full 10 with ease and continued to write until asked to stop. Each person had their own reality, likely shaped by their own experiences, processing, and beliefs about the life they had lived to date. Pondering the question of what it means to be human is necessary when it comes to constructively regarding the impacts of trauma.

Consider the multitude of people you've known throughout your life—strangers, community members, acquaintances, friends, family, the man at the bus stop you see every day. . . and most importantly yourself. You may think of some of these people with fondness and admiration and others with either indifference, confusion, or perhaps with a level of disdain. Some of these people may share similarities such as appearance, dialect, values, and more, but none of them are exactly alike. Even identical twins are distinct from one another, whether it be mannerisms, likes/dislikes, temperament, and so on.

Just as people are all unique and different, their experiences with and reactions to trauma are also different. Some people can seemingly tolerate immense amounts of stress, such as miscarriages, natural disasters, or relationship ruptures with little to no impact on their daily routines such as sleeping, eating, and functionality. Others seem to have a much lower stress threshold, losing the capacity to engage in the same daily life activities such as the aftermath of what some would view as less disturbing events such as lost car keys, brief conflict with a friend, or waking up to an empty container of coffee creamer in the refrigerator. Understanding trauma means to understand what feels safe and regulated for one person, can be experienced as unsafe, dysregulating,

"

and even traumatic to another. We are all unique, so expecting all people to experience a distressing event in the same way is not realistic.

Trauma impacts have been researched, conceptualized, and explored throughout the centuries. As a common human experience, the primary and secondary impacts of trauma continue to be a point of concern and interest for many. Trauma can be relentless and ruthless at times, stemming from acts of commission such as something tragic that happened, like violence, natural disasters, sexual assault, illness, loss, poor living conditions, abuse, or witnessing something horrific. Likewise, it can result from acts of omission or something that didn't happen—missing out on something that didn't happen that needed to, such as neglect, or not getting essential needs met during critical times of development. Regardless of whether the individual is healing from what did or didn't happen, the trauma impact can be very powerful.

Consider the voice of "Becca" as she explains the impacts of trauma (Becca is a fictional client comprised of multiple client experiences)—I'm always exhausted. My body aches. I wake up all night long, just staring at the ceiling for hours until I finally fall asleep. Since the rape, I'm numb "down there." I've turned into a raging bitch, yelling at my husband and kids over nothing. I feel angry just looking at them. They're so needy. Spoiled brats lately. No one understands how hard this is for me. All of my friends left. They weren't really friends anyway. I can literally taste his nasty smell one hundred percent of the time. When I close my eyes, I can see his face clear as day. It's been over a year already. I can't do this anymore. I can't even button my pants now. I've gained so much weight. I literally hate my life. It'd be easier to be dead than to live my life now.

Becca's voice is one of many that speaks for the masses that have suffered in the throes of trauma. She is experiencing the impacts of trauma: disrupted sleep, numbness in the pelvic area, irritability, explosiveness, decreased stress tolerance, flashbacks, heightened senses, social engagement, fluctuations in weight, and suicide ideation. Trauma is impacting her family, clientele, society, her own sense of safety and self, and ultimately her world. This could be and has been statements from many of the clients I have worked with who are struggling with the impacts of trauma.

As a trauma focused therapist, I've learned about case studies and seen pictures of when bruises would reoccur during reprocessing from decades prior, as the body was re-experiencing the traumatic event, or pattern of events. Trauma can feel excruciating and miserable, changing neural pathways in the brain to be conducive to survival states. Trauma impacts rationale, relationships, and functionality with feelings of shame, helplessness, and hopelessness, much like a tornado erratically spinning around destroying whatever is in its path. It's important to distinguish between what trauma is and what it is not. Not everyone who experiences extreme distress is traumatized. What is merely unsettling to some, can be traumatizing to another. As people, we have varying thresholds of what our system can handle before the internal alarm system is activated. Trauma can impact life in seemingly unrelated ways, leaving individuals, families, and communities perplexed, wondering about the roots of issues, not knowing the connection to trauma.

One of my young adult clients watched her mother die a violent death at a young age. Since her mother's death, she has developed an addiction to exercise. At first glance, one could view her addiction as dedication to her health. Unfortunately, exercise consumed her thoughts, took up much of her waking hours, caused her to develop injuries, lose relationships, and limited her capacity to go to work. Dr. Gabor Mate's definition of addiction would propose that my client could not slow down or stop on her own accord (2022). She recognized her focus on exercise as problematic but felt powerless to change. During her mother's funeral, my client overheard someone say "I wish she would've taken better care of her physical health. Perhaps this could've been prevented." The links can be nearly unidentifiable, leading to the felt sense of defectiveness. Sometimes something as seemingly insignificant as a well-meaning comment or misperception during a stressful time can greatly impact one's mental and physical health problems, causing one to feel shameful for what is happening inside of the nervous system. Perhaps one of the biggest impacts is feeling shameful for being human.

In the chapters of this book, there is a trove of psychotherapeutic insights from experienced and knowledgeable clinicians in the field of mental health who have committed their personal and professional lives to helping the traumatized, working as clinical psychologists and psychotherapists, developing and teaching trainings, writing books, creating therapeutic tools, participating in suicide awareness campaigns, and more. They are in the metaphorical trenches working with traumatized individuals and providing robust therapeutic approaches such as Sandtray Therapy, EMDR Therapy, Play Therapies (TraumaPlay™, Digital Play Therapy™, Attachment Centered Play Therapy, AutPlay® Therapy), Expressive Therapy, Neurofeedback, Brainspotting, and other modalities that have the potential necessary to heal trauma.

Therapy can improve, and in many cases, save lives. Trauma creates emotional wounds that can be felt in the body, and trauma-focused therapy can often heal trauma wounds. However, the type of therapy is secondary in importance to the safety and connectedness found in a healthy therapeutic relationship—a strong therapeutic relationship is at the core of all effective therapy. Otherwise, the nervous system may go into defense states to protect the person, causing therapy to be ineffective and possibly more traumatizing.

To this end, Dr. Bessel van der Kolk (2015) describes the big challenge of treating trauma in therapy as helping people live in bodies that don't feel safe, especially in the being. Without safety, even the most powerful type of therapies, as the ones listed above, will be ineffective.

The intention of this book is to inform you about various impacts of trauma with beams of hope for healing throughout. The impacts of trauma do not need to be a life sentence of misery and suffering. Perhaps every person reading this book can pose the following personal question, "What is at least one way I can support a global paradigm on the truths of trauma?" Some may decide to educate others on the importance of safety and connection, with the intent to debunk the common belief that the pain can be punished away. Others may wish to provide a more direct approach such as meeting the basic needs of traumatized people through food, shelter, and physical safety. As you read this chapter, you will better understand the impacts of trauma on individuals, specific groups, and societies. It is imperative that therapists conceptualize the impacts as they work with clients processing such powerful experiences.

## REFERENCES

Maté, G., & Maté, D. (2022). *The myth of normal: Trauma, illness, & healing in a toxic culture*. Avery (Penguin Random House).

Van der Kolk, B. A. (2015). *The body keeps the score: Brain, mind, and body in the healing of trauma*. Penguin Books.

# Foreword

When I started graduate school in 1965, at Washington University in St. Louis, to pursue a PhD in Clinical Psychology, there were few options for mental health professionals to understand and treat trauma compared to today. A half-century ago, there were studies of shell shock and combat neuroses primarily related to soldiers in combat from the two world wars. However, the study of post-traumatic stress disorder (PTSD) as we now know it through a myriad of writings and frequent teaching workshops in the mental health field was lacking. Yet, in the mid-60s, a time when the Vietnam War was creating mounting casualties, including psychiatric disorders, the young veterans coming back from the war arrived in great numbers on an acute unit of John Cochran V.A. Hospital where I was assigned part of the time that I served a 4-year traineeship and internship.

The situation was acute and called for state-of-the-art trauma treatment at a time in the mental health field when there was sparse knowledge base to draw upon and few trauma treatment programs that were available especially compared to now. Prior to the adoption of PTSD in the third edition of the Diagnostic and Statistical Manual (DSM-III,1980), the classification was Traumatic War Neurosis. At that time, psychiatrists applied the diagnosis only to adults who had experienced traumatic events. It was not until the publication of the fourth edition of the DSM (DSM-IV) in 1994 that the psychiatric field recognized PTSD as a diagnosis for children and adolescents. Since then, research has continued to develop our understanding of PTSD in children and improve methods for diagnosing and treating this condition in younger populations.

DSM-III (1980) described several symptoms and behavioral abnormalities commonly associated with PTSD. These include depression, anxiety, increased irritability linked with sporadic and unpredictable explosions of aggressive behavior, impulsivity, substance use disorders, suicidal actions, occupational impairment, and interference with interpersonal relationships (Boman, 1985). I remember vividly the fear I experienced as a young psychology trainee in the psychiatric wards of John Cochran V.A. Hospital when a veteran would erupt in a sudden, unpredictable explosion of rage and aggressive behavior that would require three or more sturdy ward attendants to subdue and restrain the patient. In our current world, we would understand such episodes as likely triggered by traumatic memories. The main library resources prior to 1965 were Abram Kardiner's (1941) *War Neuroses: Their Psychological and Clinical Aspect's*, Roy Grinker and John Spiegel's (1945) *The Traumatic Neuroses of War*, and Charles S. Meyers' (1941) *Shell Shock and its Lessons*. These texts written after World War I and World War II provided important insights rooted in psychanalytic theory into the clinical features of traumatic war neurosis. It was on the bedrock of these careful observations and the analytic treatment of post-war veterans that later advances in theory and treatment developed.

Among the best-known researchers on PTSD in the past 50 years include Judith Herman, Bessel van der Kolk, Edna Foa, and Bruce Perry. Other seminal contributors include Daniel Siegel, Allan Schore, Glenn Saxe, Judith Cohen, Anthony Mannarino, and Esther Deblinger among others. These researchers have conducted extensive studies on the dynamics of trauma, PTSD symptoms, and effective treatment strategies for PTSD.

A major appeal of this book, in addition to its focus on a wide variety of impacts resulting from trauma, is the three editors. Each of them, Jessica Stone, Robert Jason Grant, and Clair Mellenthin, is widely known in the play therapy field and for their writings and creative work in the field. All three are experienced clinicians who know firsthand the challenges and rewards of treating trauma in the field. The editors selected chapter authors well-qualified to cover an original and interesting array of topics capturing the impacts of trauma, including to the editors' credit a chapter on the impact on the therapist. Importantly, the book contains an excellent chapter on self-care as well. The impacts of trauma may be quite apparent while others are more subtle, but all involve enduring suffering that observers should never minimize or trivialize.

PTSD is a severe mental illness affecting both children and adults globally. Although the symptoms of PTSD can be debilitating, the good news is that researchers and treating clinicians are developing new treatment options, including play therapy, trauma-focused cognitive behavioral therapy, and eye movement desensitization and reprocessing (EMDR) therapy. The capable authors of this book describe an even newer treatment for child trauma, virtual reality (VR). The primary focus of this book is the impacts of trauma since there are abundant writings focused on the contributing factors that cause trauma in both adults and children. This is an essential exploration because trauma can have short-term effects but often longer-term impacts as well. It is my conviction that the acute symptoms of PTSD, which may resolve in the first 90 days after trauma exposure, do not begin to convey the major impact of interpersonal trauma. This is clearly the case in chronic or complex trauma when abusers inflict interpersonal trauma (consisting of physical or sexual abuse, neglect, or witnessing domestic violence) repeatedly sometimes throughout the child's developmental years. The impact of such deliberatively inflicted trauma, often by family members or caregivers whom the child once trusted, may rupture their sense of trust, making it difficult to repair because of the betrayal the child feels. For years or decades after, the victim of complex trauma may fear intimacy and closeness and without effective treatment the suffering can extend far beyond the acute symptoms, such as intrusive images, nightmares, and startling reactions. I will briefly describe three of the better known as well as a new innovative treatment for child trauma below.

## TRAUMA-FOCUSED COGNITIVE BEHAVIORAL THERAPY

Trauma-focused cognitive behavioral therapy (TF-CBT): This is an evidence-based treatment approach that shows effectiveness to reduce trauma symptoms in children. It combines cognitive behavioral techniques with trauma-specific interventions.

## PLAY THERAPY

Play therapy is a form of therapy frequently used for children with PTSD. Play therapy involves the use of toys, games, fantasy, imagination, and symbolic communication. Therapists encourage children to use play to work through their trauma and emotions. An advantage of play therapy is that children can use the symbolism and metaphors of play to regulate the distance or closeness to the traumatic material. The child is in control of the pacing thus keeping therapy a safe place.

## EYE MOVEMENT DESENSITIZATION AND REPROCESSING THERAPY

Eye movement desensitization and reprocessing (EMDR) therapy is a form of therapy that involves using eye movements, sounds, or tapping to help individuals process traumatic memories. It is a widely used treatment for PTSD in adults, and recent research has demonstrated that it can also be effective in children.

## VIRTUAL REALITY THERAPY

Virtual reality (VR) is a computer-generated environment that can simulate sensory experiences. VR therapy for PTSD involves exposing individuals to virtual environments that are like their traumatic experiences. While this is a novel approach, the research thus far is promising.

## CONCLUSION

This book discusses recent developments and innovations in the treatment of PTSD in children, including CBT, play therapy, EMDR therapy, and VR therapy. Most importantly, it discusses a wide range of impacts that trauma has on children and families. The treatments presented in this book have shown promising results in reducing the symptoms of PTSD in children. Future research should focus on improving the methods and techniques of these therapies, making them more accessible and affordable to children worldwide. Child trauma significantly impacts the lives of children, and it is essential that we continue to seek new and innovative ways to treat it. This book is an important contribution toward that aim.

**David A. Crenshaw, PhD, ABPP, RPT-S,** Author, Chief of Clinical Services, Children's Home of Poughkeepsie, Licensed and Certified Clinical Psychologist, Fellow of the American Psychological Association

# Introduction

CLAIR MELLENTHIN and JESSICA STONE

Trauma surrounds us, transcending geographical boundaries and lines of intersectionality. It pervades every corner of the world, impacting individuals, communities, and society at large. Through various mediums such as television, social media, and podcasts, our consciousness can become immersed in a deluge of stories depicting any number of atrocities occurring globally. We actively seek out this information, exposing ourselves collectively to primary and secondary forms of trauma. However, our perception tends to focus primarily on the individual experience, disregarding the profound impact on those who share their space within our collective memory.

Trauma often tricks our brain into thinking *I am completely alone* and *No one could ever begin to imagine the pain and anguish I am experiencing*. This leads to isolation and a closing off from relationships; when ironically, relationships are crucial for healing (despite often being the source of pain). The aftermath of trauma and its impact on interpersonal relationships, social support networks, and the broader environment are frequently overlooked, silenced, or disregarded. Yet, this omission suppresses a crucial component of the trauma narrative. Without acknowledging these effects, constructing a coherent story for the individual's healing becomes challenging. As Van der Kolk aptly states, "Being traumatized means continuing to organize your life as if the trauma were still ongoing - unchanged and immutable – as every new encounter or event is contaminated by the past." (2015, p. 53). When all parties involved in a traumatic experience begin to withdraw and isolate themselves, concealing their pain, shame, and secrets, the very bonds that are meant to foster healing and connection become fragmented and strained. The act of closing off from one another contributes to the fraying of these bonds, thus hindering the potential for healing and growth.

## THE IMPACT OF TRAUMA

Our understanding of traumatic experiences includes those that involve exposure to real or threatened physical and/or sexual violence, death, serious injury, and being witness to these events (American Psychiatric

Association, 2022). Large-scale natural disasters, war, famine, racism, migration, immigration, and global pandemics often form the eye-grabbing headlines of the day. These global and community-based traumas impact our lives in complex mechanisms throughout the many systems and subsystems we interact with daily. Large-scale disasters, such as war, natural calamities, and climate change, place significant strain on vital resources that a society requires for its survival. These encompass essential aspects such as healthcare, economic security, and environmental safety. The overwhelming impact of such disasters exacerbates the challenges in ensuring the availability and effectiveness of these critical resources.

Our present global interconnectedness has mitigated the isolating effects that previous generations faced when conflicts were limited to their immediate communities. A prime illustration of this is the ongoing war in Ukraine, which presently affects grain availability and prices worldwide. Consequently, this has led to food insecurity in various African nations, declining stock prices in the United States, fuel shortages throughout Europe, and, with the latest assault, water insecurity across Ukraine and neighboring countries. The looming threat of a potential nuclear disaster adds a layer of risk that would impact the entirety of Europe (United Nations, 2023).

The interconnected nature of our world underscores the intricate relationships between multiple ecosystems, revealing how they mutually influence and impact one another. This interconnectedness extends to the lives of all individuals within these intersecting subsystems. Even though traumas may arise at local or community level, the profound effects ripple through the lives of those directly or indirectly exposed. It is crucial to recognize both the visible and hidden dimensions of trauma in order to support those most affected in forging a path toward healing. By acknowledging the overt and covert impacts of trauma, we can foster a comprehensive understanding and offer meaningful assistance to those on their healing journey.

## IMPACT ON THE INDIVIDUAL

Trauma can manifest either in an individual's isolated experience or within the intricate framework of a dynamic or systemic context. Regardless of the manifestation, the impact of trauma on the individual is profound and far-reaching. At the individual level, trauma can disrupt cognitive processes, distort emotional regulation, and impair the development of a coherent sense of self (van der Kolk, 2015; Weisner, 2020). The consequences of trauma on the individual's mental, emotional, and physical well-being can be enduring, necessitating sensitive and comprehensive interventions to promote healing and recovery.

Within the individual, a complex network of neural clusters forms cognitive and emotional connections to the present traumatic event, as well as any past experiences. These interconnected neural pathways contribute to the profound impact of the trauma on the individual's psyche. Moreover, the connections between the individual and the various systems they are a part of, including current relationships and intergenerational influences, compound and complicate the overall trauma experience. The interplay between these elements further shapes the individual's perception and response to the trauma, highlighting the intricate and multifaceted nature of its effects.

Regardless of the duration, repetitive nature, or uniqueness of the traumatic experiences, individuals may perceive the trauma as a separate entity from others, internally navigating its unique impact (Lynn, 2022). Traumatic experiences can encompass both objective and subjective characteristics, as defined by the Substance Abuse and Mental Health Services Administration (SAMHSA, 2015). Objective characteristics refer to tangible and observable elements, while subjective characteristics pertain to internal processes, such as emotional responses. The nature and components of the event(s), an individual's personal characteristics, the specific type of trauma, and sociocultural factors all contribute to how an individual is affected by the traumatic experience (Lynn, 2022).

## IMPACT ON THE FAMILY SYSTEM

Covert or "invisible" forms of trauma, which occur within interpersonal relationships, have a profound and lasting impact on an individual's life trajectory and development. Coined by Herman (1992), the term "complex trauma" describes the repetitive experience of chronic physical, sexual, and emotional abuse within the parent–child or family relationship. When this chronic complex trauma persists across generations within a family, it is known as intergenerational transmission of trauma (Fitzgerald et al., 2020). The traumatic experiences are passed down from one generation to the next through their interactions.

Childhood victimization involving multiple forms of abuse impairs neurodevelopment, relational learning, and overall physical and emotional well-being. This cycle of chronic and complex trauma leads to the development of anxious and insecure attachment styles, depressive symptoms, and complex post-traumatic stress disorder (C-PTSD) symptoms, such as dissociation and affect dysregulation, in adulthood (Spinazzola et al., 2021).

These interpersonally experienced, covert traumas have a profound impact on individuals, shaping their development and leaving an indelible mark on their lives. Recognizing and understanding the effects of complex trauma is crucial for promoting healing and providing appropriate support to individuals who have endured such experiences.

Herman (1992) notes that when unresolved childhood trauma persists throughout a lifetime, it can manifest within interpersonal relationships even if the physical or sexual violence has stopped. A parent who is traumatized may utilize negative coping skills when they feel stressed and overwhelmed such as yelling, inconsistent and harsh parenting, physical punishment, isolation, non-communication, or other maladaptive child-rearing techniques that they in turn learned from their parents. This leads to a cycle of attachment trauma that is further ingrained and reinforced with each generation (Spinazzola et al., 2021).

It is highly likely that individuals will encounter one or more traumatic events throughout their lifetime (Papero, 2017). Furthermore, discovering that a loved one or a person in a close relationship has experienced such an event can also be profoundly traumatic (Russin & Stein, 2022). Extensive research indicates that the aftermath of abuse and trauma is exceptionally challenging and distressing, not only for the primary victim but also for those connected to them within the relationship. Russin and Stein's comprehensive literature review on the systemic impact of trauma reveals that individuals within formal support networks, including friends, family members, and significant others of sexual assault survivors, often experience feelings of anger directed toward God, the perpetrator, the victim, and society as a whole (2022). Additionally, they note the presence of caregiver burden and factors of secondary traumatic stress, which significantly affect mental health and interpersonal relationships. It is important to acknowledge that being a supportive family member to a trauma survivor has a notable impact on one's psychological well-being. Common experiences reported in Russin and Stein's research include feelings of guilt, helplessness, anger, self-blame, depression, and even suicidal ideation.

Russin and Stein (2022) also found that there are significant markers for resiliency and healing within family systems following tragedy and trauma. In families where there are high levels of self-efficacy, relationship quality, and relationship communication, the effects of anxiety and depression decrease. Additionally, families who emphasize expressiveness and cohesion tend to have the lowest levels of psychiatric symptomology.

## A SYSTEMIC FOCUS

Viewing trauma through a systemic lens helps us to make sense of how the traumatic experiences of our lives shape our view of ourselves, our relationships and connections within and between the many broader systems we interact with, and the greater world around us. Understanding how trauma impacts and influences these same systems and subsystems is crucial in beginning to develop a pathway toward holistic and integrative healing. It is our hope that this book will help bridge the gap in understanding the many areas of intersectionality that a traumatic experience impacts.

## REFERENCES

American Psychiatric Association (1980). *Diagnostic and statistical manual of mental disorders* (3rd ed.). American Psychiatric Publishing.

American Psychiatric Association (2022). *Diagnostic and statistical manual of mental disorders, fifth edition, text revision (DSM-5-TR)*. American Psychiatric Association.

Boman, B. (1985). Post-traumatic stress disorder (traumatic war neurosis) and concurrent psychiatric illness among Australian Vietnam veterans: A controlled study. *Journal of the Royal Army Medical Corps, 131*, 128–131.

Fitzgerald, M., London-Johnson, A., & Gallus, K. L. (2020). Intergenerational transmission of trauma and family systems theory: An empirical investigation. *Journal of Family Therapy, 42*, 406–424.

Grinker, R. R., & Spiegel, J. P. (1945). *The traumatic neuroses of war.*

Herman, J. (1992). *Trauma and recovery.* Basic Books.

Kardiner, A. (1941). *War neuroses: Their psychological and clinical aspects.*

Lynn, C. (2022). Understanding and impact of trauma. *Journal of Forensic Psychology, 7*(211).https://www.walshmedicalmedia.com/open-access/understanding-and-impact-of-trauma.pdf

Meyers, C. S. (1941). *Shell shock and its lessons.* Manchester University Press.

Papero, D. V. (2017). Trauma and the family: A systems-orientated approach. *Australian and New Zealand Journal of Family Therapy, 38*, 582–594.

Russin, S. E., & Stein, C. H. (2022). The aftermath of trauma and abuse and the impact on the family: A narrative literature review. *Trauma, Violence, and Abuse, 23*(4), 1288–1301.

SAMHSA (2015). Trauma-informed care in behavioral health services: Kap keys for clinicians. https://store.samhsa.gov/sites/default/files/d7/priv/sma15-4420.pdf

Spinazzola, J., van der Kolk, B., & Ford, J. D. (2021). Developmental trauma disorder: A legacy of attachment trauma in victimized children. *Journal of Traumatic Stress, 34*, 711–720.

United Nations (6 March, 2023). *One year of the war in Ukraine leaves lasting scars on the global economy.* https://www.un.org/en/desa/one-year-war-ukraine-leaves-lasting-scars-global-economy

van der Kolk, B. (2015). *The body keeps the score: Brain, mind, and body in the healing of trauma.* Penguin Books.

Weisner, L. (2020). *Individual and community trauma: Individual experiences in collective environments. Illinois Criminal Justice Information Authority Center for Violence Prevention and Intervention Research.* https://www.researchgate.net/publication/343236178_Individual_and_community_trauma_Individual_experiences_in_collective_environments

# Section I

# The Impacts of Trauma

## CHAPTER ONE

# A Foundation for Human Connection and the Impact of Trauma

FIONA HILL

A natural response when accidentally touching a hot surface is to pull away quickly in order to prevent getting burned. The same can be said for humans when they face adversity in the context of connection and relationships. Whether in the form of lashing out in anger, running away in fear, or collapsing in overwhelm, true to its duty of protection, the nervous system quickly shifts into a shield mode when it detects danger within one's body, environment, and/or relationships (Dana, 2018). This chapter will focus on three key areas related to the innate need for human connection: exploration of history and theoretical foundations, analyzing psychological and sociological frameworks, and their role in gaining an understanding of the impact trauma has individually and collectively.

The autonomic nervous system (ANS) consists of three states: ventral vagal, sympathetic, and dorsal vagal. The ventral vagal state provides acknowledgment of engagement and felt safety, while the sympathetic state is one of high alert, and the dorsal vagal state indicates collapse and hibernation. All of these are necessary and fluid states of being (Dana, 2018). Whatever state the nervous system is in at any given moment is necessary for self-preservation within that experience. Subsequently, each state is not meant to last indefinitely, and humans are not meant to function in complete independence of one another; rather, one's best existence happens within healthy interdependent

*Trauma Impacts: The Repercussions of Individual and Collective Trauma*, First Edition.
Edited by Jessica Stone, Robert J. Grant, and Clair Mellenthin.
© 2024 John Wiley & Sons, Inc. Published 2024 by John Wiley & Sons, Inc.

relationships. The way in which one navigates life does not rely on the notion that adversity will never happen; rather, it acknowledges the need for available opportunities in which to experience a sense of safety through connectedness and relationships. Fluidity through each state with some level of felt safety allows for increased integration and resilience. Adversely, being stuck in any of the three states can alter one's worldview and perception of reality; thus, impacting how humanity relates to their environment and each other (Perrotta, 2020).

While the experience of the global COVID-19 pandemic was far from pleasant and indeed traumatic in its local, national, and global impact, clinicians and researchers have gained insights and made observations that may not have occurred otherwise. One notable insight has been the broader and deeper understanding of the benefits of using technology to improve personal emotional quality, engagement, actualization, and connectedness (Riva et al., 2020). Society has been "forced" to widen its lens with which both the building and maintaining of human relationships are considered. With the exponential growth of accessibility to technology and its use in connecting people all over the world in ways that were previously only imagined, opportunities for ongoing research will be beneficial for years to come. Even though the modalities that one experiences connection internally and interpersonally may change, the basis for the need for a relationship is not new. From the beginning of time, our "brains were wired for connection" (Lieberman, 2013, p. 9).

Through exploring history and theories of human connection, the groundwork can be laid for a purposeful and intentional discussion of relational connection. Having this foundation is essential when building research, practice, and conversations related to healthy relationships, as well as those disrupted by adverse experiences in childhood and adulthood. Understanding the psychological and sociological frameworks of human connection provides the necessary structure in which we can more easily conceptualize both human needs and human behavior. The risk lies in analyzing the power of connection through each of these lenses in isolation; however, when developed through an integrated perspective, the impact of adverse experiences on "felt-safety" for individuals and society can be more deeply understood—in hopes of deeper healing for all.

## CONNECTION DEFINED

The word "connection" can seem to be an arbitrary term with shallow existence. Merriam-Webster (n.d.) defines *connection* as "a relation of personal intimacy (as of family ties)." However, forming and maintaining connections is anything but a straightforward process and reaches far beyond the familial connection. To fully integrate what it means to connect with yourself and others, it is important to consider the etymology of the word. *Connect* came into English in the 15th century, derived from the Latin "conectere" meaning "join together," which in its time was formed from "com," meaning "together," and "nectere," meaning "to tie or bind" (MacMillan Dictionary Blog, 2017). With the understanding that the term *connection* is an umbrella term for the process of understanding one's world through building relationships, other terms that may be used synonymously are intimacy, attachment, bond, and attunement.

## NEUROSCIENCE AND CONNECTION

Within the research of neuroscience, it is difficult to pinpoint one primary contributor. The work of Drs. Bessel van der Kolk, Daniel Siegel (Interpersonal Neurobiology), Stephen Porges (Polyvagal Theory), and others has been paramount in understanding the brain science of relationships and how adverse events can disrupt the inner workings of the nervous system; therefore, disrupting one's ability to form and maintain healthy connections. Interpersonal Neurobiology primarily focuses on neural integration of the nervous system in order to produce regulation and felt safety (Siegel, 2020), while the Polyvagal Theory focuses on "repatterning the ways the autonomic nervous systems operate when the drive to survive competes with the longing to connect with others" (Dana, 2018, p. 3).

Forming attachment and connection is universal across lifespan and cultural contexts, regardless of the quality of care in infancy (Bowlby, 1988; Naeem et al., 2022). Whether positive or negative, imprints are stored in the human mind and body through neural networks—shaping both interpersonal and intrapersonal interactions. These impressions become the lens through which relationships are not only viewed but also approached and interacted with (van der Kolk, 2014).

In understanding connection and the human drive to be in relationship with others, an important question is "Why?" *Why do past experiences directly impact relational engagement with the present world?* If we examine the human need for connection and attachment through a biological perspective and, more specifically, a neurobiological lens, it easily makes sense. How human connections are disrupted through traumatic experiences changes the focus of one's nervous system. This change can often result in physical, mental, and emotional symptomology (van der Kolk, 2014).

## THEORETICAL AND HISTORICAL FOUNDATIONS

In considering the evolution of the field of psychology over the past several decades, it makes sense that thoughts, understanding, perspectives, and practical applications of foundational theories have shifted; however, the foundational human need for connection and the impact of disruption without repair remain. This insight highlights, rather than minimizes, the importance of viewing individual and collective trauma experiences through both theoretical and historical lenses. Strong historical and theoretical foundation provides a launching pad for current and future clinical work. Furthermore, a sound theoretical orientation provides the clinician with a framework from which to base therapeutic interventions. While there is a plethora of theoretical frameworks that can be discussed, for the sake of brevity, only a few will be addressed in this chapter.

## THEORY OF HUMAN MOTIVATION

Maslow's Theory of Human Motivation, or Maslow's Hierarchy of Needs (1943), provides an introductory scope into human connection needs. Early in his career, Maslow (1943) proposed that everyone has five basic needs: physiological (food, water, sex), safety (from danger), social (love, affection, and belonging), esteem (high esteem of themselves and others), and self-actualization (doing things one is meant to do).

The main tenet of Maslow's work is that each need builds upon the other, and to achieve self-actualization, all five needs must be met. He writes,

> Human needs arrange themselves in hierarchies of pre-potency. That is to say, the appearance of one need usually rests on the prior satisfaction of another, more pre-potent need...Also no need or drive can be treated as if it were isolated or discrete; every drive is related to the state of satisfaction or dissatisfaction of other drives. (Maslow, 1943, p. 372)

While Maslow (1943) describes these needs as a hierarchical system and identifies physiological needs as the most important contributor to one's homeostasis, he also acknowledges that the meeting of these needs can be fluid. Maslow (1943) acknowledges in his paper *A Theory of Human Motivation* that other intrinsic needs are not accounted for, which also provide physiological homeostasis, such as "sensory pleasures (taste, smells, tickling, stroking) which are probably physiological, and which may become the goals of motivated behavior" (p. 372). Maslow's inquisition led him to later expound on the concept of self-actualization. Rather than it being the "end all, be all" and the idea that one has "arrived" once self-actualization has been achieved, there is transcendence or the peak experience in which an individual has greater ability to identify greater independence within themselves and their surrounding environment. This peak experience includes what Maslow termed the cognition of being or B-cognition (Maslow, 1962). One's ability to experience B-cognition allows for greater space to "hear and listen" (Maslow, 1970); thus,

B-cognition is an important element in fostering compassion and empathy for others during individual and collective trauma experiences.

Maslow's work presents interesting dichotomies that most certainly warrant a more in-depth examination of his original writings, particularly the cognition of being and peak experience. Through laying the groundwork for more contemporary theories, he provided a launching pad for current and ongoing research on the innate human need for connection and relationship, both within and outside of the individual experience.

## General Systems Theory

The concept of systems is not new and can be traced back to philosophers from as early as the 1920s: Leibniz (natural philosophy), Nicholas of Cusa (coincidence of opposites), Paracelus (mystic medicine), and Vico and ibn-Kaldun (vision of history as a sequence of cultural entities), among others; however, it is Ludwig von Bertalnaffy's work, in the 1940s, that is credited for bringing these and other concepts together into what is known as General Systems Theory, or GST (von Bertalanffy, 1968). The theory was born out of his desire for there to be "unity" among the sciences—a general framework organizing foundational concepts that can be generalized across science disciplines (von Bertalanffy, 1968). Montuori (2011) summarized the systems theory approach in this manner:

> The term systems approach is widely used as an umbrella for concepts and ideas drawn from general system theory, cybernetics, chaos theory, and complexity theory. The term covers an approach to inquiry that is not limited to one discipline and proposes a new way of thinking about the world focusing on interconnected, interdependent, dynamical systems, rather than parts that can be isolated from the whole. (p. 414)

Consider the operation of a vehicle. While it is feasible that some parts are not vital to its direct operation, there are some that can pose danger if left unattended. For instance, properly working brake lights are necessary, particularly when driving at night or in adverse weather conditions to alert other drivers of a pending stop. The vehicle is operational without working brake lights; however, malfunctioning brake lights could potentially disrupt the system's overall safety. When there is a shift in one area, the entire system experiences the effects. Within this one example, there are multiple mechanical and human systems at work simultaneously. Like the vehicle analogy, social systems operate both interdependently and intradependently. If there is to be recognizable growth in systemic healing from the impacts of trauma, understanding human interaction and connectedness through a culturally relevant systemic lens is important.

While von Bertalanffy (1968) addresses the application of GST regarding social sciences, in part, by its very design, further research and exploration was necessary to apply his foundational work more specifically to the field of social science. As a result, there is a multiplicity of theoretical branches stemming from Bertalanffy's work, adding another layer to understanding human connection (von Bertalanffy, 1968).

## FAMILY SYSTEMS THEORY

Family Systems Theory (FST) is among many stemming from GST (Fleming, 2018) and is an important contribution to understanding human connection as it relates to the individual and collective impact of adverse events, primarily developed by Murray Bowen (Kerr & Bowen, 1988). "The core objectives are decreasing the anxiety or tension within a system by observing family patterns, facilitating awareness of how the emotional system functions, and increasing levels of autonomy and differentiation among the members of the system, while remaining emotionally connected to the intensity of a significant relationship system" (Kerr & Bowen, 1988). While simplified into three primary objectives, looking through an FST lens is anything but simple. There are eight interlocking key components that make up patterns of relationship: nuclear family emotional system, differentiation of self, triangles, cutoff, family projection process, multigenerational process, sibling position, and emotional process in society (Gilbert, 2013). For detailed explanation of these components, see *The Eight Concepts of Bowen Theory* (Gilbert, 2013).

While foundational in the pursuit of understanding relationship dynamics, connectedness, and human behavior, FST is not without flaws. A valid critique is the limits regarding the original theory's ability to include diverse family, gender, socioeconomic, and cultural perspectives. There has been an overt shift in recent years to expand the lens of foundational theories such as FST to be more inclusive of cultural differences that make up contemporary family systems. Erdem and Safi (2018) propose an integration of the Cultural Lens Approach (CLA), Family Change Theory (FCT), and Multicultural Perspective to expand the theory's applicability with modern families while also maintaining the authentic purpose of FST—decreasing chronic anxiety within a family system and increasing differentiation within the system.

The CLA, based on the work of Hardin et al. (2014), includes five steps in evaluating the cultural validity of psychological theory. When followed, these steps lead to relevant evaluation questions that can highlight necessary shifts toward inclusivity (Erdem & Safi, 2018; Hardin et al., 2014) for a comprehensive explanation.

Çiğdem Kağıtçıbaşı's primary contribution through FCT was a study conducted evaluating the value of children (VoC) and intersectionality within the family system. Her research found that motives for having children differed, depending on cultural context and socioeconomic status; therefore, promoting different family models and self-identities (Erdem & Safi, 2018).

The contribution of Carter and McGoldrick (1988) to the integration of a more culturally inclusive application of FST pulls in the multigenerational and cross-cultural experiences of chronic anxiety and the implications for the family system (Erdem & Safi, 2018).

At its core, an integrated systems approach provides another vital launching pad to a deeper understanding of trauma's impact on human connection cross-culturally.

## Attachment Theory

Given that attachment relationships are systemic in nature, it is not surprising that key concepts related to both systems and attachment theories are similar. Both consider the relationship processes (Ng & Smith, 2006), and the goal is system regulation. John Bowlby began his research in 1950 and developed his theory of attachment based on the parent–child dyad system (Bowlby, 1988). His work based on this research, *Maternal Care and Mental Health*, was published in 1951 (Bowlby, 1988, p. 35), and he is known as the "father of attachment theory" (Mooney, 2010). His work, along with others such as Mary Ainsworth, is based on the thought that the detached nature in children he worked with was a result of early separation from family members (Bowlby, 1988). As noted by Carol Mooney, the early research from Bowlby indicates that attachment was primarily centered around the relationship between a mother and her infant, while more contemporary research includes both parents and other significant adults (Mooney, 2010). Given the amount of trauma experiences in which children lose one or both parents, this shift toward including other caregivers is both a necessary and powerful one.

Historically, in its healthiest form, attachment has been thought to serve as a protective link between the mother and her infant (Bowlby, 1988; Mooney, 2010). A few key principles of Bowlby's attachment theory (1988) include thoughts on intimacy, attachment dynamics, attachment categories, and attachment across the lifespan (1988).

One's potential to thrive developmentally and emotionally largely depends on the opportunity to experience and build connection around a healthy sense of intimacy through identifying and seeking those who provide felt safety, also known as a secure base (Bowlby, 1988). Bowlby and Ainsworth developed four child attachment categories, which help understand the parent–child relationship and how adults connect and interact with each other more fully. These categories include secure, avoidant, anxious, and disorganized attachment styles (Holmes, 2015). When a child grows into an adult, the way they interact with the world does not automatically change. In fact, the opposite is true. A child's past experiences directly influence how the same adult experiences the present world (Siegel, 2020).

The way connection-seeking is navigated during adverse experiences is determined by the individual and collective attachment patterns developed. In her book *Attachment Centered Play Therapy*, Clair Mellenthin describes this navigation process as being on a continuum that fluctuates between chaotic and secure attachment, rather than fitting into a specified attachment "box" (2019). She states,

> It is important to note that no one is 100% securely attached or. . .100% chaotically attached or unattached. We all land somewhere in the middle or tend to fluctuate within the same scope of the spectrum in most of our relationships. (p. 5)

A language of continuum offers the necessary flexibility for not only acknowledging but also understanding the innate connection needs of others at any given moment; therefore, increasing the ability to offer more compassionate, empathic, and attuned connections during adverse experiences.

Relationships are like a dance. The ability to be fully immersed in an activity without being fully aware of one's surroundings, all the while experiencing a sense of intrinsic enjoyment from the activity is known as being in a state of "flow" or "in the zone." Flow, or the optimal experience, was first developed by psychologist Mihaly Csikszentmihalyi to make sense of his traumatic experiences during WWII and in pursuit of the meaning of happiness. In alignment with systems and attachment theories previously mentioned, flow theory (Csikszentmihalyi, 1990) views the human experience from both individual and collective perspectives—addressing the pursuit of happiness internally (within oneself) and externally (relationship with others). For optimal experiences to occur within relationships, experiencing feelings of safety is key. Adverse experiences affect one's feeling of safety, and as a result, impact the internal and external flow of relationships (Dana, 2018).

## TRAUMA'S IMPACT

A variety of scenarios are easily identifiable as trauma, such as sexual violence, domestic violence, and war, to name a few; however, there are situations that occur that may not be as easily identifiable. An adverse event, or trauma, can happen to anyone at any time, and the way in which it is experienced is subjective (Csikszentmihalyi, 1990; Dana, 2018); therefore, the human perspective and perception of safety and flow are subjective. Furthermore, one individual's experience of a traumatic event may not be a shared experience with others. There are three key factors that determine recovery from adverse experiences: having a sense of felt safety that produces connection, calmness, and hope; access to physical and emotional support; and the ability to experience self-empowerment (Csikszentmihalyi, 1990; Gusak, 2017).

Prolonged exposure to severe early childhood trauma, especially in the parent–child relationship, impacts the child's brain development and disrupts the ability to adapt to life stressors in a healthy manner. One of the first indicators of a disruption in a caregiver–infant relationship is the presence of anxiety (Naeem et al., 2022). Ruptured attachment during times of extreme stress often results in a caregiver's inability to help reduce the infant's level of stress hormones through co-regulation in times of threat. (Naeem et al., 2022).

While some impacts of traumatic caregiver–infant relationships are readily apparent in childhood, others appear later into adolescence and extend further than post-traumatic stress disorder (Ford, 2018). Adolescence is an important transitional period in which the neural pathways supporting executive functioning are still developing (Ford, 2018). Consequently, it stands to reason that navigating a traumatic experience would have a significant impact on regulation, impulsivity, and social relationships (Ford, 2018). Further, those who experience early childhood trauma, and in adolescence, are at a greater risk of re-victimization (Ford, 2018).

Indicators of childhood trauma presenting later in adulthood can be even more obscure, such as low self-esteem, depression, substance abuse, and self-isolation (Downey & Crummy, 2022). In 1998, Felitti et al. published the *Adverse Childhood Experiences* (ACE) study. It was a two-wave study originally conducted from 1995 to 1997 by the CDC in partnership with Kaiser (Felitti et al., 1998). In this study, the researchers were "assessing, retrospectively and prospectively, the long-term impact of abuse and household dysfunction during childhood on the following outcomes in adults: disease risk factors and incidence, quality of life, health care utilization, and mortality" (Felitti et al., 1998, p. 246). The results concluded that there is, indeed, a strong correlation between the amount of one's ACE and multiple risk factors: smoking, severe obesity, physical inactivity, depressed mood, suicide attempts, alcoholism, any drug abuse, parenteral drug abuse, a high lifetime number of sexual partners, and a history of having a sexually transmitted disease for death in adults (Felitti et al., 1998). All of which directly and indirectly impact experiences of connectedness, attunement, and attachment throughout the lifespan.

Trauma can also impact an entire group or society. Collective trauma is "a group-level cataclysmic, tragic experience that is reproduced through co-constructed discourse" (Hirschberger, 2018). Within this collective experience, there are many individual experiences—each one subjectively based on current knowledge and past experiences. Collective trauma is often thought to be an experience within a larger context, such as natural disasters, mass shootings, and social injustices. These are certainly tragic collective experiences that affect feelings of connectedness. However, collective trauma can be experienced on a much smaller scale—within family systems, friendship groups, and religious congregations, to name a few. Realistically, any group experience of the same traumatic event is collective.

## CONCLUSION

One function of the brain is to continuously analyze and assess for safety within the body, environment, and relationships through the ANS (Dana, 2018; Porges, 2017). This analysis and assessment process is an attempt to provide understanding and direction. Traumatic experiences intensify this function. When words are insufficient or unreachable, emotions are the avenue of understanding. In fact, they are foundational to attachment throughout the lifespan; furthermore, collaboratively sharing these experiences forms attachment that supports and strengthens connectedness. On the contrary, when there is a lack of opportunity to share experiences in a supportive environment, disenfranchisement is the result (Stanley et al., 2021).

Given that all humans are wired for connection, the feelings of loneliness, detachment, and isolation have the potential to impact all areas of an individual and society. While it is important to know the negative implications of disrupted connections, it is equally important to acknowledge the hope of healing that lies within what we are learning about the innate human need for connection and how to therapeutically connect with those who are entrusting their care to the helpers. "A more inclusive, cohesive, and connected modern approach is listening, understanding (to the best of our abilities), and affirming lived experiences that diverge from our own. Instead. . .we must meet others where they are to enhance our collective perspective" (Altvater, 2023, p. 40). As an individual member of a collective community navigating life's experiences, listening with curiosity and hearing with compassion is vital.

## REFERENCES

Altvater, R. A. (2023). *Perspective: Contemplating the complexities of our realities*. Creative Publishing.

von Bertalanffy, L. (1968). *General system theory: Foundations, development, applications*. Braziller: Penguin.

Bowlby, J. (1988). *A secure base: Parent-child attachment and healthy human development*. Basic Books.

Carter, E. A., & McGoldrick, M. (1988). *The changing life cycle: A framework for family therapy*. Gardner Press.

Csikszentmihalyi, M. (1990). *Flow: The psychology of optimal experience*. HarperCollins Publishers.

Dana, D. (2018). *The polyvagal theory in therapy: Engaging the rhythm of regulation*. W.W. Norton & Company.

Downey, C., & Crummy, A. (2022). The impact of childhood trauma on children's wellbeing and adult behavior. *European Journal of Trauma & Dissociation, 6*(1), 100237. https://doi.org/10.1016/j.ejtd.2021.100237

Erdem, G., & Safi, O. A. (2018). The cultural lens approach to Bowen family systems theory: Contributions of family change theory. *Journal of Family Theory & Review, 10*(2), 469–483. https://doi.org/10.1111/jftr.12258

Felitti, V. J., Anda, R. F., Nordenberg, D., Williamson, D. F., Spitz, A. M., Edwards, V., Koss, M. P., & Marks, J. S. (1998). Relationship of childhood abuse and household dysfunction to many of the leading causes of death in adults: The Adverse Childhood Experiences (ACE) Study. *American Journal of Preventive Medicine, 14*(4), 245–258. https://doi.org/10.1016/s0749-3797(98)00017-8

Fleming, W. M. (2018, February 22). Family systems theory. *International Encyclopedia of Marriage and Family*. encyclopedia.com https://www.encyclopedia.com/social-sciences-and-law/sociology-and-social-reform/sociology-general-terms-and-concepts/family-systems-theory.

Ford, J. D. (2018). Complex trauma and developmental trauma disorder in adolescence. *Adolescent Psychiatry, 7*(4), 220–235. https://doi.org/10.2174/2210676608666180112160419

Gilbert, R. M. (2013). *The eight concepts of bowen theory: A new way of thinking about the individual and the group*. Leading Systems Press.

Gusak, N. (2017, January 1). *Mental health and psychosocial support: Resilience vs trauma*. Ukma. https://academia.edu/79149978/Mental_Health_and_Psychosocial_Support_Reslilience_vs_Trauma

Hardin, E. E., Robitschek, C., Flores, L. Y., Navarro, R. L., & Ashton, M. W. (2014). The cultural lens approach to evaluating cultural validity of psychological theory. *American Psychologist, 69*(7), 656–668. https://doi.org/10.1037/a0036532

Hirschberger, G. (2018). Collective trauma and the social construction of meaning. *Frontiers in Psychology, 9*. https://doi.org/10.3389/fpsyg.2018.01441

Holmes, J. (2015). Attachment theory in clinical practice: A personal account. *British Journal of Psychology, 31*(2), 208–228. https://doi.org/10.1111/bjop.2009.100.issue-1

Kerr, M. E., & Bowen, M. (1988). *Family evaluation: An approach based on Bowen theory*. W.W. Norton.

van der Kolk, B. (2014). *The body keeps the score: Brain, mind, and body in the healing of trauma*. Penguin Books.

Lieberman, M. D. (2013). *Social: Why our brains are wired to connect*. Crown.

MacMillan Dictionary Blog. (2017). *Connected*. https://www.macmillandictionaryblog.com/connected

Maslow, A. H. (1943). A theory of human motivation. *Psychological Review, 50*(4), 370–397. https://doi.org/10.1037/11305-004

Maslow, A. H. (1962). *Toward a psychology of being*. Martino Fine Books.

Maslow, A. H. (1970). *Religions, values and peak-experiences*. Viking Press.

Mellenthin, C. (2019). *Attachment based play therapy*. Routledge.

Merriam-Webster. (n.d.). Connection. *Merriam-Webster.com*. https://www.merriam-webster.com/dictionary/connection

Montuori, A. (2011). Systems approach. *Encyclopedia of Creativity*, 414–421. https://doi.org/10.1016/b978-0-12-375038-9.00212-0

Mooney, C. G. (2010). *Theories of attachment*. Redleaf Press.

Naeem, N., Zanca, R. M., Weinstein, S., Urquieta, A., Sosa, A., Yu, B., & Sullivan, R. M. (2022). The neurobiology of infant attachment-trauma and disruption of parent–infant interactions. *Frontiers in Behavioral Neuroscience, 16*. https://doi.org/10.3389/fnbeh.2022.882464

Ng, K.-M., & Smith, S. D. (2006). The relationships between attachment theory and intergenerational family systems theory. *The Family Journal, 14*(4), 430–440. https://doi.org/10.1177/1066480706290976

Perrotta, G. (2020). Psychological trauma: Definition, clinical contexts, neural correlations and therapeutic approaches. *Current Research in Psychiatry and Brain Disorders, 1*(1), 1–6.

Porges, S. W. (2017). *The pocket guide to the Polyvagal Theory: The transformative power of feeling safe*. W.W. Norton & Company.

Riva, G., Mantovani, F., & Wiederhold, B. K. (2020). Positive technology and covid-19. *Cyberpsychology, Behavior, and Social Networking, 23*(9), 581–587. https://doi.org/10.1089/cyber.2020.29194.gri

Siegel, D. J. (2020). *The developing mind: How relationships and the brain interact to shape who we are*. Guilford Press.

Stanley, B. L., Zanin, A. C., Avalos, B. L., Tracy, S. J., & Town, S. (2021). Collective emotion during collective trauma: A metaphor analysis of the COVID-19 pandemic. *Qualitative Health Research, 31*(10), 1890–1903. https://doi.org/10.1177/10497323211011589

CHAPTER TWO

# Dimensions of Deprivation

RACHEL A. ALTVATER

Trauma is life-altering, as it shifts perspective and adjusts one's way of being. While varied in frequency, intensity, and duration, traumatic encounters are an increasingly prevalent human experience. Many individuals, families, and communities have been and continue to be confronted with situations that challenge their sense of safety. The impacts are diversified, as trauma lies within the eye of the beholder. In other words, while traumatic instances may be overtly categorized as such, the perceptions within each individual's unique position and the subsequent reactions are ultimately what influence the ongoing perspective of self, others, and the world (Altvater, 2023).

This chapter explores the impact of actual, perceived, or the fear of deprivation following a single incident or complex traumatic encounter(s). When we experience trauma, our perception of the world around us is adjusted through the lens of that trauma. If our basic needs are compromised, we form the presumption that those needs could become compromised again. Our nervous system and other self-preservation mechanisms attempt to protect us for survival, so we experience some degree of hypervigilance and connect to the threat. This degree and manner of connection vary person-to-person, but a common thread for humans is a prolonged fear of obtaining fundamental necessities and persisting through current and future endangerments. Gaining insight into the ramifications of trauma and deprivation encourages resolutions that are grounded in effective

*Trauma Impacts: The Repercussions of Individual and Collective Trauma*, First Edition.
Edited by Jessica Stone, Robert J. Grant, and Clair Mellenthin.
© 2024 John Wiley & Sons, Inc. Published 2024 by John Wiley & Sons, Inc.

methods for combatting recurrent traumatization, not only for individuals and communities but for generations to come.

## OVERVIEW

Experiencing deprivation is typically dangerous and terrifying. Deprivation is not having access to basic necessities or lacking something one needs. With an absence of core essentials for survival, living beings are placed in an extremely vulnerable situation that ultimately brings about perceptions, and perhaps a reality, of the potential cessation of life. This shift in the perspective of safety and security impacts humans on a psychobiological level, inevitably altering the ongoing navigation of their lives.

### NERVOUS SYSTEM UNDERSTANDINGS

The autonomic nervous system (ANS) is a primary biological system that activates during and following traumatic and deprivation encounters. The ANS is a component of the peripheral nervous system (PNS), which functions to relay messages between the brain and the body (UC San Diego Health, n.d.). The PNS consists of sensory, autonomic, and motor neurons. Sensory neurons connect the brain and spinal cord to the senses, namely the skin. Autonomic neurons are responsible for involuntary functions, including heart rate, digestion, blood pressure, and other essential physical reactions. Motor neurons link the brain and spinal cord to muscles for stimulation (UC San Diego Health, n.d.). The primary focus of further exploration and understanding will be on the autonomic neurons within the ANS.

The ANS comprises the sympathetic, parasympathetic, and enteric nervous systems. The sympathetic nervous system (SNS) manages a fight–flight–freeze–fawn response, which is a self-defense reaction to confront, run from, remain paralyzed by, or cave into danger as a means of survival. The increase in cortisol, adrenaline, blood flow, and oxygen use allows the body to have the necessary energy to act accordingly (Anderson, 2022). The parasympathetic nervous system activates a resting state to assist the body in returning to equilibrium. The enteric nervous system focuses on digestion and nutrient absorption (Anderson, 2022). Trauma and high-stress confrontations most often trigger the SNS.

The SNS operates automatically, without conscious thought. Simply put, it responds without waiting for the brain to carefully dissect and process information. When it receives any indication of concerning stimuli, prior to the brain forming a cohesive thought and direction, the body rapidly responds to prepare itself to act as a method of self-preservation. The time it takes to form a logical conceptualization of what is occurring could be a matter of life and death, so the body acts prior to receiving clarity; there is often no initial distinction between real and perceived threats; rather, all stimuli are assumed to be real threats to offer the body the chance to react accordingly in an instant.

Once there is SNS arousal, the body preserves the memory of the encounter for future preparation. Connecting these nervous system concepts to deprivation, when there is an experience where a basic need is left unmet, the brain and body become aware of this reality and either consistently experience it or assume the possibility of it recurring. If the body is in a constant state of concern for the unfulfillment of needs, continual chemical and electrical danger messages will cycle through the ANS; the brain and body remain stagnant in believing that danger is looming ahead because the body is informing the brain that there is something that is the cause for concern. This feedback loop is the cause of long-standing disturbances.

## Human Needs

Traumatic experiences commonly disrupt and deprive people of a host of basic and higher-order human needs. As aforementioned, deprivation is varied and complex due to the degree and one's perception of a single incident or complex traumatic encounter(s). Different people will respond in different manners to similar experiences due to variations in perspectives (Altvater, 2023). Areas of deprivation due to unmet or compromised needs include but are not limited to the following: sleeping, eating, daily functioning, relationships, memory and other cognitive functioning, access to sufficient care, socioeconomic deficits, homelessness, and loss.

Dr. Abraham Maslow (1943), a renowned and revered American psychologist, theorized a motivational hierarchy of human needs. He identified five stages of needs—physiological, safety, love and belonging, esteem, and self-actualization. Psychological needs are essential for core human functioning and include air, water, food, shelter, sleep, clothing/warmth, and sex/reproduction. Safety needs pertain to personal security, health, and access to resources. Love and belonging are the needs that focus on a sense of close connection with others. Esteem needs relate to respect for oneself, a healthy self-concept, and a feeling of accomplishment. The self-actualization need is reaching one's fullest potential and seeking personal growth and peak experiences. Dr. Maslow visually presented these in the configuration of a pyramid, with physiological needs at the base, self-actualization at the peak, and all identified stages progressing in order in between. Ultimately, he expressed that the needs at the foundation of the pyramid are to be satisfied prior to obtaining subsequent needs.

Dr. Maslow's (1943, 1962, 1987) hierarchy is divided into deficiency and growth needs. The deficiency needs consist of the first four levels, and the growth need, also referred to as being need, is the fifth peak level. Deficiency needs occur as a result of deprivation. Dr. Maslow believed that deficiency served as a motivator to fulfill needs, and that the longer a person is unable to attain the needs, the stronger the desire to meet them. He explained that the lower-level needs must be sufficiently met prior to progressing forward. When the deficiency needs are attained, people are able to focus more on personal growth. Progress is often interrupted or fluctuates due to challenges with adequate fulfillment of lower-level needs.

Dr. Maslow (1943) delineated that perspectives of needs shift depending on the needs that are sufficiently or insufficiently met. The following is his salient explanation of this concept:

> when a need has been satisfied for a long time, this need may be underevaluated [sic]. People who have never experienced chronic hunger are apt to underestimate its effects and to look upon food as a rather unimportant thing. If they are dominated by a higher need, this higher need will seem to be the most important of all. It then becomes possible, and indeed does actually happen, that they may, for the sake of this higher need, put themselves into the position of being deprived in a more basic need. We may expect that after a long-time deprivation of the more basic need there will be a tendency to reevaluate both needs so that the more pre-potent [sic] need will actually become consciously prepotent for the individual who may have given it up very lightly. Thus, a man who has given up his job rather than lose his self-respect, and who then starves for six months or so, may be willing to take his job back even at the price of losing his a [sic] self-respect. (p. 388)

Deprivation inescapably alters one's focus of attention and subjective reality.

## HISTORICAL CONTEXT

Trauma was reportedly first examined in the psychological literature during the last decades of the 19th century. Increased interest and attention resurfaced during World War II, when Dr. Abram Kardiner (1941), an American psychiatrist and psychoanalytic therapist, published his book, *The Traumatic Neuroses of War*, which discussed his treatment of World War I veterans. Trauma research re-emerged as an important area of exploration again in the late 1970s during the Vietnam War and women's movement (van der Kolk, 2000). While the focus of investigations waxed and waned and ongoing clarity was not obtained throughout time, trauma has clearly remained a consistent aspect of human history.

It is confidently postulated that the impact of trauma far exceeds the literature. Both modern and historical writing acknowledges an astronomical number of human atrocities, natural disasters, other crises, and threats to safety. As expressed by van der Kolk (2000):

> The human response to psychological trauma is one of the most important public health problems in the world. Traumatic events such as family and social violence, rapes and assaults, disasters, wars, accidents and predatory violence confront people with such horror and threat that it may temporarily or permanently alter their capacity to cope, their biological threat perception, and their concepts of themselves. (p. 7)

Traumatic experiences and subsequent impacts are timeless; the primary difference between the past and present is our refined understanding.

A major focus of historical trauma deprivation research was related to the detrimental developmental impacts of grave neglect toward institutionalized children. It was discovered that through the early 20th century, these children often encountered serious ramifications, including mental, emotional, behavioral, physical, and relational challenges, severe developmental and cognitive delays, and death, due to insufficient care, fulfillment of basic needs, stimulation, and caretaker relationships (Gunnar & Reid, 2019). This and the later research taught us that a lack of basic needs during this highly impressionable time leaves a lasting imprint.

Overall, there is a dearth of historical research on deprivation, likely due to the sporadic and centralized nature of trauma research and the shift in cultural perspectives on what is considered a traumatic event. For example, in ancient times, children were viewed as property. Practices such as infanticide, child mutilation, severe punishment, and child labor were common and accepted in most cultures. It was not until the early 20th century that there was a major shift of protection for abused and neglected children (Thomas, 1972). With greater recognition of trauma symptoms and impacts and an intentional shift to trauma-focused care, greater discoveries are being made and clarity is attained about trauma and deprivation.

## PSYCHOLOGICAL IMPACT

Scholars and researchers have shown increased interest over the past several decades in investigating the intricacies of trauma and deprivation, so the field's compendium has widely expanded in a relatively short time frame. One area of particular interest is the psychological impact of deprivation. Adverse experiences in various contexts, including but not limited to maternal deprivation (Bowlby, 1969), early socio-emotional deprivation (Eluvathingal et al.,2006; McDermott et al., 2013), economic deprivation (Knifton & Inglis, 2020; Waters & Moore, 2001), deprivation in regions affected by conflict (Hammoudeh et al., 2021), and relative deprivation (lacking the same standard of living as those in close proximity or that they are accustomed to; Chen, 2015), consistently show that deprivation results in psychological distress and mental and physical unwellness. Collectively, these findings support the notion that when people lack actual and/or perceived fundamental needs, the mind and body respond in a dysregulated manner. Insufficient resources and a lack of necessary human experiences result in an inability to fully function, feel safe and secure, and receive ample nourishment.

Another area of heightened interest is the impact of early trauma and deprivation on neural development. The formation of all aspects of our being begins in early childhood, and each experience ultimately shapes the brain and influences burgeoning perspectives and ongoing relationships with self, others, and the world (Altvater, 2023). Through refined analysis, it was discovered that due to "the developing brain anticipat[ing] certain kinds of environmental input at certain times, substantial deviations from what is needed and anticipated can compromise brain and behavioral development" (Zeanah & Sonuga-Barke, 2016, p. 1099). Researchers also proposed that deprivation is a distinct pathway to psychopathology through certain brain circuits (McLaughlin et al., 2014) and different types of traumas impact the targeted brain regions (Teicher & Samson, 2016). Thus, trauma and deprivation directly influence the structure and function of the brain. Alterations in "normal" or expected brain development will inevitably result in lasting psychological consequences.

## RELATIONAL DISRUPTIONS

People thrive in spaces where they are able to rely on and connect with the collective. The human species has advanced significantly throughout time due to the ability to share information and resources; humans transformed into an interconnected global community heavily reliant on one another to access and obtain basic needs. When each person plays a role within a specified group or community, the system functions seemingly well, and the members are generally satisfied. However, when there is a fight for resources or needs that are insufficiently met by others, the perspective about relationships and one's place within the group shifts.

Physical, emotional, or social deprivation consequently disrupts relationships. Damaging relational experiences, whether from early childhood experiences (e.g., attachment disturbances) or through peer or community interactions (e.g., bullying, discrimination, and inclusivity), result in the formation of a core belief, or conception in one's mind, that this is a typical experience, and others will operate similarly. People are more likely to be standoffish or disengage from interactions with others if they do not serve them in a beneficial manner.

As previously denoted, when a person lacks basic necessities and their ANS is activated, they are likely to operate from a space of survival. If there is a lack of connection and a threat to the accessibility of resources, they might operate in a manner to attain and/or protect whatever they can for self-preservation. When there is a perception that others cannot be trusted or relied upon, they are more likely to be viewed as unsupportive, undependable, and perhaps unsafe. Fending for oneself becomes a default for protection. Detachment from others then further perpetuates deprivation experiences and magnifies psychological consequences. Social isolation is found to lead to adverse health consequences, including depression, sleep disturbances, executive functioning challenges, cognitive decline, impaired physical health, and premature death (Novotney, 2019).

## Detachment from Self

Not only does deprivation disconnect people from others, but it also detaches people from themselves. The initial conception of self in early childhood is adapted from what is learned about the self from others; modeled behavior provides a blueprint for ongoing interactions and expectations. So, in the case of early deprivation, the lasting impression of self is likely to be rooted in experiences and messages that evoke feelings of inadequacy. When internalizing this information, people might feel self-rejection and unworthiness in having their needs met. This perspective flavors ongoing thoughts, feelings, and engagement with the self (Altvater, 2023). Psychological symptoms, including self-injurious behaviors, dissociations or detachment from self, low self-esteem, self-doubt, and a lack of self-trust and self-compassion, are all common precipitants of trauma and deprivation, likely due to these damaging views of self (Center for Substance Abuse Treatment [US], 2014).

Dr. Matthew Bowker (2016) explores the concept of detachment from self-following trauma and deprivation in his book, *Ideologies of Experience: Trauma, Failure, Deprivation, and the Abandonment of the Self*. He explains that there are discourses and attitudes that work against the development of the self, which he refers to as "ideologies of experience." He proposes that ideologies of experience following trauma and deprivation result in identifying with the experience's "objects" and abandoning the self. People split their experiences from their own thoughts and engage in introjection, unconsciously adapting the ideas of others. This becomes a stagnant, compulsive, and repetitive behavior that discourages creative and purposeful action and results in an increasingly solidified rejection of the self.

## CONTEMPORARY (21ST CENTURY) ISSUES

Prior to the digital era, there were limited avenues for receiving information. Centuries ago, it took an extended period of time to travel on foot or by animal to deliver messages to others in distant areas. Now, people are deeply interconnected and inundated with information from all corners of the world in mere seconds. While there is a plethora of benefits to modern accessibility, the rapid and constant consumption of tragic and horrific news flashes takes its toll on the psyche. Bearing witness to others' traumas and then receiving little to no break until the next piece of heart-wrenching information is shared can be mentally, emotionally, and physically taxing. This experience often enhances anxiety, depression, and vicarious trauma. There is also an intensification of polarization, where people are socially pressured to choose a side in unrelenting conflicts, which results in unceasing strife and further division. This immense fear and tension result in actual or perceived deprivation for many.

One of the most prevalent contemporary global deprivation experiences emerged during the coronavirus (COVID-19) pandemic (World Health Organization, n.d.). A scarcity mindset, the pervasive feeling of not having enough, contributed to perceived and actual deprivation. People protected themselves and those closest to them; they worked to safeguard those in their innermost circle(s), trying to retain as many resources as possible for protection and survival. Emptying grocery stores, hoarding toilet paper, and struggling to obtain necessities or other resources for protection resulted in many people defaulting to self-preservation mode.

The unfortunate reality is that despite the collective resources and wealth to sustain all people, there are many who lack crucial supplies. Those in underdeveloped and war-ridden countries or territories, those living in poverty or experiencing homelessness, those struggling to afford basic necessities due to the rise in cost and availability, and vulnerable people (e.g., children, elders, and those who are disabled) who receive subpar care are in a constant state of distress and uncertainty. Deprivation is a serious unresolved matter that impacts more people globally every single day.

## FUTURE RAMIFICATIONS

Younger generations initially encounter and adopt life through older generations' perspective lenses. Messages of affliction are shared, creating a legacy of trauma and deprivation, commonly referred to as intergenerational trauma (DeAngelis, 2019). Dr. Elena Cherepanov examined how survivors' initial reactions to an event may affect future generations. As recounted by DeAngelis (2019),

Living under such difficult, oppressive circumstances, [Dr. Cherepanov] surmises, can lead parents to formulate fear-based "survival messages" that they pass on to their children and grandchildren—ideas like "Don't ask for help—it's dangerous." While the messages may have initially helped people stay alive, in the present they are often irrelevant and may even increase people's interpersonal vulnerability. (Transmission mechanisms Section)

Insufficiently addressing the manner in which people collectively consume and manage trauma and deprivation will lead to prolonged and intensified psychological issues. People are generally unsure how to navigate overpowering emotional experiences, so they remain in a space of pain and suffering when they do not seek additional support. It would behoove people to increase insight and awareness into what is being consumed, how it impacts them, and methods of coping. Otherwise, the trauma and deprivation experiences will remain an all-consuming experience that ripples outward and will recurrently be passed on to others.

Compassion for and genuine safe connection to others is an essential avenue that has the potential to mitigate the repercussions of trauma and deprivation. Compassion is a deep feeling for and desire to relieve another's suffering. Research suggests that compassion enhances emotions when confronted with distressing experiences (Klimecki et al., 2013) and aids psychological health and well-being (Jazaieri et al., 2013). When people experience healing through compassionate connections, concerns for ongoing deprivation are decreased, as there is reassurance of probable support. As a result, it is more likely for the pained legacy of trauma to shift toward a more united and cohesive perspective of others. Much needs to be provided for and/or worked on between those who have deep-rooted trauma and deprivation experiences to nurture default danger and skeptical nervous system responses.

## CONCLUSION

The core of our being is rooted in survival. Living creatures are biologically programmed to spread their seeds for repopulation and the sustainability of the species. This foundational drive is responsible for the brain and body's extreme responses when confronted with real or perceived threats or when the fulfillment of basic needs becomes compromised. Being deprived of human essentials poses a threat to the safety of the individual and the longevity of the collective, resulting in an assortment of mental, emotional, and relational complications.

Deprivation is a life-altering experience, completely adjusting one's way of perceiving and existing within the world. When needs are routinely met, people are more likely to confidently proceed with the expectation that this will continue to occur; little to no thought goes into meeting these needs. When traumatic encounters cease regular or sufficient obtainment of basic needs, automatic responses shift focus to safely and swiftly seeking those needs. These experiences then further program the body's neural network and leave lasting psychobiological impressions.

Reintegration into a "normal" routine once there is greater consistency in the fulfillment of needs is inevitably met with skepticism. The rewiring of neuronal chemical and electric messages programs the brain and body for future re-encounters and tumultuous possibilities. Reshaping of internal structures and connections directly influences all future external engagements in some form. Deprivation is a terrifying human encounter that requires lifelong conscious efforts to manage, not only for self but also for future generations that are likely to vicariously absorb the messaging and lifestyles that accompany it.

## REFERENCES


Altvater, R. A. (2023). *Perspective: Contemplating the complexities of our realities*. Creative Publishing.

Anderson, A. (2022). *Autonomic nervous system: What to know*. WebMD. https://www.webmd.com/brain/autonomic-nervous-system-what-to-know

Bowker, M. H. (2016). *Ideologies of experience: Trauma, failure, deprivation, and the abandonment of self*. Routledge.

Bowlby, J. (1969). *Attachment and loss, vol. 1: Attachment. Attachment and loss*. Basic Books.

Center for Substance Abuse Treatment (US) (2014). *Trauma-informed care in behavioral health services*. (Report No. (SMA) 14-4816). Substance Abuse and Mental Health Services Administration. https://store.samhsa.gov/sites/default/files/d7/priv/sma14-4816.pdf

Chen, X. (2015). Relative deprivation and individual well-being: Low status and a feeling of relative deprivation are detrimental to health and happiness. *IZA World of Labor*, 140. https://doi.org/10.15185/izawol.140

DeAngelis, T. (2019, February). The legacy of trauma. *Monitor on Psychology, 50*(2), 36. https://www.apa.org/monitor/2019/02/legacy-trauma

Eluvathingal, T. J., Chugani, H. T., Behen, M. E., Juhász, C., Muzik, O., Maqbool, M., Chugani, D. C., & Makki, M. (2006). Abnormal brain connectivity in children after early severe socioemotional deprivation: A diffusion tensor imaging study. *Pediatrics, 117*(6), 2093–2100. https://doi.org/10.1542/peds.2005-1727

Gunnar, M. R., & Reid, B. M. (2019). Early deprivation revisited: Contemporary studies of the impact on young children of institutional care. *Annual Review of Developmental Psychology, 1*, 93–118. https://doi.org/10.1146/annurev-devpsych-121318-085013

Hammoudeh, W., Mitwalli, S., Kafri, R., Lin, T. K., Giacaman, R., & Leone, T. (2021). The psychological impact of deprivation in regions affected by conflict: A multilevel analysis of a cross-sectional survey in the occupied Palestinian territory. *Lancet (London, England), 398*(Suppl 1), S29. https://doi.org/10.1016/S0140-6736(21)01515-4

Jazaieri, H., Thupten Jinpa, G., McGonigal, K., Rosenberg, E. L., Finkelstein, J., Simon-Thomas, E., Cullen, M., Doty, J. R., Gross, J. J., & Goldin, P. R. (2013). Enhancing compassion: A randomized controlled trial of a compassion cultivation program. *Journal of Happiness Studies, 14*(4), 1113–1126. https://doi.org/10.1007/s10902-012-9373-z

Kardiner, A. (1941). *The traumatic neuroses of war.* National Research Council. https://doi.org/10.1037/10581-000

Klimecki, O. M., Leiberg, S., Lamm, C., & Singer, T. (2013). Functional neural plasticity and associated changes in positive affect after compassion training. *Cereb Cortex, 23*(7), 1552–1561. https://doi.org/10.1093/cercor/bhs142

Knifton, L., & Inglis, G. (2020). Poverty and mental health: Policy, practice and research implications. *BJPsych Bulletin, 44*(5), 193–196. https://doi.org/10.1192/bjb.2020.78

van der Kolk, B. (2000). Posttraumatic stress disorder and the nature of trauma. *Dialogues in Clinical Neuroscience, 2*(1), 7–22. https://doi.org/10.31887/DCNS.2000.2.1/bvdkolk

Maslow, A. H. (1943). A theory of human motivation. *Psychological Review, 50*(4), 370–396. https://doi.org/10.1037/h0054346

Maslow, A. H. (1962). *Toward a psychology of being.* D. Van Nostrand Company.

Maslow, A. H. (1987). *Motivation and personality* (3rd ed.). Pearson Education.

McDermott, J. M., Troller-Renfree, S., Vanderwert, R., Nelson, C. A., Zeanah, C. H., & Fox, N. A. (2013). Psychosocial deprivation, executive functions, and the emergence of socio-emotional behavior problems. *Frontiers in Human Neuroscience, 7*, 167. https://doi.org/10.3389/fnhum.2013.00167

McLaughlin, K., Sheridan, M., & Lambert, H. (2014). Childhood adversity and neural development: Deprivation and threat as distinct dimensions of experience. *Neuroscience and Biobehavioral Reviews, 47*, 578–591. https://doi.org/10.1016/j.neubiorev.2014.10.012

Novotney, A. (2019, May). The risks of social isolation. *Monitor on Psychology, 50*(5), 32.

Teicher, M. H., & Samson, J. A. (2016). Annual research review: Enduring neurobiological effects of childhood abuse and neglect. *Journal of Child Psychology and Psychiatry, 57*, 241–266. https://doi.org/10.1111/jcpp.12507

Thomas, M. P. (1972). Child abuse and neglect part 1: Historical overview, legal matrix, and social perspectives. *North Carolina Law Review, 50*, 293–349. https://scholarship.law.unc.edu/nclr/vol50/iss2/3/

UC San Diego Health. (n.d.) *About peripheral nervous system (PNS).* https://health.ucsd.edu/specialties/neuro/specialty-programs/peripheral-nerve-disorders/pages/about-peripheral-nerves.aspx#:~:text=The%20peripheral%20nervous%20system%20is,to%20the%20central%20nervous%20system.

Waters, L. E., & Moore, K. A. (2001). Coping with economic deprivation during unemployment. *Journal of Economic Psychology, 22*(4), 461–482. https://doi.org/10.1016/S0167-4870(01)00046-0

World Health Organization. (n.d.). *Coronavirus disease (COVID-19) pandemic.* https://www.who.int/emergencies/diseases/novel-coronavirus-2019.

Zeanah, C. H., & Sonuga-Barke, E. J. (2016). Editorial: The effects of early trauma and deprivation on human development—From measuring cumulative risk to characterizing specific mechanisms. *Journal of Child Psychology and Psychiatry, and Allied Disciplines, 57*(10), 1099–1102. https://doi.org/10.1111/jcpp.12642

## CHAPTER THREE

# Impact on Abilities for Personal Self-Care

MARY ANNE PEABODY

Self-care: two little words connected and separated by a hyphen. Metaphorically, the hyphen serves as a symbolic representation of the "in-between space" where two phenomena exist. Often when the word self-care is applied to the construct of trauma, it is at the level of the individual, although trauma can also occur at the familial or systemic level. In this chapter, self-care will be explored at the level of the individual, the prime unit of self-care. However, it is important to note that individual-level trauma-based treatment involves work on the "self" and assistance or "help" from others. Therefore, the hyphenated space between these two little words connotes both individualism and collectivism; separation and connection.

Trauma, whether it is a one-time event, continuous, historical, or systemic, causes deep psychological disruption. The impact of trauma often involves a fragmented sense of self that is experienced physically, cognitively, psychologically, and spiritually, further impacting one's relationship with the world (Frewen et al., 2020; Maté, 2022). Trauma can create disconnections with the body, emotions, and the ability to live in the present moment, which potentially robs individuals of the desire to engage in self-care. When an individual's sense of self is deeply shaken, they may face existential challenges when processing difficult emotions and thoughts, so the capacity to engage in self-care thoughts or actions may feel inconceivable.

For our purposes, self-care will be referred to as a combination of behaviors and practices that lead to survival, healing, and health (Baker & Denyes, 2008). Such practices and behaviors involve a constellation of activities that encompass eating a well-balanced diet, engaging in exercise or physical activity, obtaining adequate rest, promoting emotional and mental health, and seeking support or assistance as appropriate (World Health Organization, 2014). Self-care refers not only to engagement in the aforementioned activities but also to a set of capacities or the emotional agency to feel compassion toward oneself (Kissil & Niño, 2017; Narasimhan et al., 2019). The literature on self-care is expansive, traversing across health promotion, disease prevention, treatment, rehabilitation, and palliative care with a variety of theories, models, and interventions generally focusing on emotional or behavioral change (Jaarsma et al., 2021).

To frame our thinking, the conceptual lens of "liminality" is used to capture the "in-between space" of trauma and its impact on self-care. The word liminal comes from the Latin root *limen*, which means threshold (Franks & Meteyard, 2007). Liminality is an experience of being "in-between" an original state and a transformed state, either spatially or temporally (Turner, 1967). When a client's trauma experience transgresses between both physical and psychological symptoms, it incurs a liminal status (Honkasalo, 2001).

Another recent example of liminality that we collectively are still experiencing as an entire society is the global pandemic. The pandemic created the "before/after experience," common to liminal time, spaces, and thinking. Depending on the personal and familial impact of the pandemic, individuals were on a liminal continuum from small stressors all the way to experiences that resulted in various levels of trauma. Conversely, the pandemic also illuminated the importance of self-care across social, emotional, and physical domains. Self-care typically requires planning, access to certain experiences, and solitude, which were in short supply during the pandemic. During the initial weeks of isolation, when many traditional activities were no longer an option, some individuals reported experiencing a disconnection with self and others; therefore, the need for creative self-care was high (Dogden-Magee, 2021).

Therefore, this conceptualization brings us to this question: Why is the concept of liminality important to therapists? The answer lies in this "in-between" space and time of transition in which the therapist can make the maximum impact on the client. The role of the mental health professional is to protect and contain the liminal spaces for clients as they progress, which often involves engaging in behaviors of self-care. As liminal experiences fuel ambiguity, confusion, and uncertainties (Beech, 2011), they paradoxically also encourage creativity, and a sense of new structures, routines, and relationships (Czarniawska & Mazza, 2003). During liminal experiences, ideas once held as certain are challenged and thrown into doubt, and although this can be disorienting, it allows a person to imagine possibilities far beyond what they may have ever been able to imagine before.

Given that trauma is pervasive across the histories of mental health clients (National Technical Assistance Center for State Mental Health Planning, 2004), understanding the interrelatedness between trauma, liminality, and self-care is vital to effective treatment. Framing the work of trauma and self-care through the prism of liminality, marked with points of transition and change, is helpful for exploring the far-reaching impact of trauma on the ability to engage in self-care, the loss of meaning, and ambivalence. Therefore, it will be important to explore the history of liminality, trauma, and self-care; the psychological impact of trauma situated in the framework of liminality; research on self-care and trauma; a brief exploration of one approach that includes self-care strategies for behavioral change; and contemporary issues. To begin the exploration, an understanding of historical context is needed.

## HISTORY

### LIMINALITY HISTORY

Liminality has both spatial and temporal dimensions. The concept of time and space in liminality was first developed in the early 20th century by Arnold van Gennep (1908) and later taken up by Victor Turner (1967). As anthropologists, van Gennep focused on individual and collective rituals (1908), and Turner expanded into human reactions (1967). Turner explored how liminal experiences shape personality and discussed how these experiences were both disorienting and growth-producing (1967). Within psychotherapy, Jungian-based analytical psychology has been deeply rooted in the ideas of liminality, seeing liminality as part of an individual's self-realization and individualization process (Jung, 1957/1960). Additionally, liminality has continued to appeal to many present-day researchers across a wide array of fields and interests, such as St. John (2008) in the field of religion, Beech (2011) in identity construction, Mackay Yarnal (2006) in aging, and McGuire and Georges (2003) in nursing and immigrant studies.

### TRAUMA HISTORY

The word "trauma" within the context of the mental health field has evolved since the 1800s when it was described as a psychic wound (Goodyear-Brown, 2010). Early researchers first described trauma by observing the short- and long-term effects on Vietnam veterans (Courtois & Gold, 2009). Simultaneously, there was an increase in public awareness of violence against women and children, with the inclusion of posttraumatic stress disorder (PTSD) in the American Psychiatric Association's (1980) *Diagnostic and Statistical Manual of Mental Disorders*, 3rd ed. (DSM-3).

As research continued and clinical debates were fueled by the curiosity of practitioners, a variety of definitions, conceptual frameworks, and classification systems evolved and expanded (Nebrosky, 2003; Shapiro & Maxfield, 2002). It became evident that the complexity of the psychobiological responses to trauma, not the actual event or experience, was where the focus points within the intervention should be situated (Briere & Scott, 2006). As Bessel van der Kolk (2014), a renowned author, researcher, and psychiatrist, shared about the multi-faceted nature of trauma:

> Trauma is not just an event that took place sometime in the past; it is also the imprint left by that experience on the mind, brain, and body. This imprint has ongoing consequences for how the human organism manages to survive in the present. (p. 21)

The devasting effects of trauma on individuals' biology are expressed in multiple ways, through vulnerable responses to a host of illnesses or addictions, including increased stress hormones, immunology difficulties, the ability to process ordinary information, and the capacity for self-regulation and self-care (van der Kolk, 2014; Maté, 2022).

## Self-Care History

The history of self-care can be traced back to primitive cultures using special foods, rituals, and shared knowledge passed from generation-to-generation (Bohart & Tallman, 1996). Later, self-care was adopted within the medical profession by doctors who wanted patients to actively participate in healthy habits and practices (Narasimhan et al., 2019). Part of the evolution history also included self-care for the practitioner. Professionals in high-risk and emotionally daunting professions, such as first responders, emergency room personnel, and professionals in the mental health fields, began to use the term for the prevention of compassion fatigue and burnout (Joinson, 1992).

Society continued to embrace self-care awareness as part of the broader context of health care and holistic well-being. People began discovering that self-care was a daily health investment, and this mindset remains relevant today. In contemporary medical practice, self-care has become very prominent as the interconnections of mental and physical health, supported by self-care attention to stress, diet, and fitness, have a strong evidentiary base of support (Maté, 2022; Ohrnberger et al., 2017; Surtees et al., 2008).

## PSYCHOLOGICAL IMPACT OF TRAUMA ON
## SELF-CARE REVISITED

If the very nature of trauma can separate an individual from their physical body, psychological feelings, and from living in the present, what brings someone to cross the liminal space to commit to caring about themselves? How do individuals create the behavioral shift in their thinking, emotions, and actions to prioritize caring for the self? How can everyday normative activities be conceptualized as small self-care steps that create a level of consistency so that caring for oneself becomes habitual? How, as therapists, can we support the healing and reconnection needed in trauma response work that honors and motivates the crossing of the liminal threshold toward health and balance? These questions are part of our reflective responsibility to better understand the liminal spaces between the trauma experience, self-awareness, self-understanding, and self-care actions.

It is important to consider this lens of liminality can be fraught with both potency and potentiality. On one side, the potency dimension exists as trauma often thwarts the individual from engaging in everyday normative activities such as seeking medical services, engaging in psychotherapy, attending familial or social activities, or celebrations such as birthdays, weddings, anniversaries, funerals, or vacations. The impact of trauma can make daily tasks and commitments feel like an uphill climb, requiring professional mental health support and purposeful interventions.

Paradoxically, liminality also holds potentiality, specifically around self-care practices. Self-care can serve as the vehicle for small movements through the liminal threshold to deeper understanding and acknowledgment of the self. Within these small movements, there are myriad benefits, holding possibilities of progressive change and lessons to be learned, if we can support our clients to become attentive students.

Understanding how self-care practices shape and influence one's "sense of self" will help both therapists and clients match treatment approaches to the specific preferences and needs of the client. Given each client has a distinctive trauma story and responds uniquely to the liminal experience of psychotherapy, assessment, and treatment approaches should be carefully matched and individualized.


## RESEARCH ON SELF-CARE AND TRAUMA

Research on re-establishing, or establishing for the first time, a sense of self has been a focus of research and treatment for trauma-related disorders for decades (van der Kolk, 2014). Overcoming the fragmentary nature of traumatic memories, increasing emotional awareness, and helping individuals with trauma reclaim their bodies and sense of self are critical components of both present- and past-centered therapies. While the various therapies around the notion of self are beyond the scope of this chapter, the following broad spectrum of researched treatments address self-care principles in various ways and is frequently cited in the trauma treatment literature: trauma-focused cognitive behavioral therapy (Deblinger et al., 2011; Mannarino & Cohen, 2017), Eye Movement Desensitization and Reprocessing (EMDR, Shapiro & Maxfield, 2002), Prolonged Exposure Therapy (PET, Foa et al., 2007), Mindfulness Therapy and mindfulness training (Boyd et al., 2018; King et al., 2016), neurofeedback (Kluetsch et al., 2014), Dialectical Behavioral Therapy (DBT, Linehan, 1993), and Acceptance and Commitment Therapy (ACT, Hayes et al., 2012).

One approach, ACT, aligns well with the conceptualization of liminality and associated self-care practices and will be briefly explored (Hayes et al., 2012). The fine-grained behavioral interpretations of ACT as a theoretical approach to trauma treatment are beyond the scope of this chapter; however, readers are encouraged to read Hayes et al. (2022) for a deeper analysis of ACT.

## ACCEPTANCE AND COMMITMENT THERAPY

ACT is an evidence-based, action-oriented treatment approach to psychotherapy that is firmly grounded in traditional behavior therapy and cognitive behavioral therapy (Hayes & Hofmann, 2021). Clients are taught several small, actionable steps nestled under the three broad domains of the therapy: mindfulness and acceptance practices, committed and valued action, and self-compassion practices. First, in behavioral terms, mindfulness and acceptance processes involve paying purposeful attention to the present moment, allowing or making space for unwanted thoughts and emotions, and relinquishing attachment to trauma-infused thoughts as if they are literal truths. Second, commitment and valued action involve making a promise to oneself about something that really matters and following through with that commitment. Third, self-compassion involves self-kindness and a willingness to acknowledge difficult thoughts and emotions without staying attached to them (Neff, 2012).

## MINDFULNESS AND ACCEPTANCE PRACTICES

Present-moment awareness can begin in the therapy session by helping clients notice what is being experienced in the "here and now." In this stage, therapists remind clients to "start small" and that "small things matter" as the key principles for action (Dindo et al., 2017). Therapists also encourage the transfer of the present-moment awareness practice into daily normative living—self-care activities that clients are already doing, such as making breakfast, showering, walking, or folding laundry, so that it constitutes no or minimal extra effort. Present-moment awareness involves purposeful attention to small things that are meaningful; for example, drinking a cup of coffee, feeling the softness and warmth of a blanket, sharing a bedtime story with their child, or a quiet moment while walking.

## Acceptance

A necessary corollary to practicing present-moment awareness is overall *acceptance*, which does not mean tolerance, endurance, or "getting used to" stressors. Rather, it refers to an awareness of, and openness to, the realization that inevitable sadness and stressors are part of the human experience. The acceptance of trauma and the emotional waves of normative life experiences are key to the tolerance of a liminal space toward health.

## Defusing from Painful Thoughts

Slowing down to notice thoughts is another strategy in this domain. By encouraging clients to take a few moments to slow down and bring curiosity to their thoughts is part of helping clients become less attached to painful or harmful thinking. In essence, this practice supports mindful awareness of, and detachment from, one's painful thoughts, such that clients are better able to notice and be influenced by the healthier cues in their environments.

## Perspective-Taking-Reflection

ACT practitioners may encourage clients, during calm moments, to reflect back—noticing patterns, antecedents to the feelings, thoughts, and corresponding behaviors. In doing so, the therapist guides the clients to mindful awareness of potentially unhelpful patterns—such as denial or avoidance of self-care. And conversely, therapists work to help clients notice and reinforce "steps that promoted the care of self," to bring these positive steps into awareness.

## Valued and Committed Actions

ACT practitioners help clients explore their values and what is important in their lives, reminding them that every moment offers a choice. By connecting with values, practitioners can hold the space necessary for clients to transform struggle and uncertainty into an opportunity to connect with what matters to them the most. Understanding values then helps clients to shift toward committed action related to caring for oneself.

Trauma can keep clients in patterns of behavior that are so ingrained they barely notice their ability or inability to choose the next steps. Thus, circling back to the previous concepts of slowing down, noticing, choosing, and starting small can bolster committed actional steps. In doing so, practitioners can help clients contribute to the creation of more helpful patterns of behavior that support engagement in what they personally value. Clients commit not only cognitively but behaviorally through actual actions of self-care.

## SELF-COMPASSION

As previously mentioned, a shaken or fragmented sense of self is often the outcome of trauma. When a sense of self is shaken, it is easy to understand that relating to ourselves with kindness and compassion or staying present and open to our pain and struggle are difficult tasks (Neff, 2012). Yet, there is ample evidence that self-compassion builds resilience (Beaumont et al., 2016; Durkin et al., 2016) and is a strong predictor of positive overall psychological health and quality of life (Baer et al., 2012; Van Dam et al., 2011). Treating oneself kindly and with compassion is synonymous with self-care.

## 21ST CENTURY FOCUS: CONTEMPORARY ISSUES AND UNMET NEEDS

Renowned physician Gabor Maté (2022) has presented a contemporary perspective that 21st-century cultural stressors are strongly impacting the collective society, and that healing cannot be hastened, but it can certainly be helped along (p. 374). He speaks to the notion that helping clients accept how things are in the present and have been in the past can provide authentic movement across the threshold to healthy grief (p. 381). Staying and supporting clients as they progress and pass through the liminal space as part of their healing journey fits with Maté's (2022) notion that healing is considered a process, not an endpoint (p. 391).

Another contemporary self-care focus has been attention given to the self-care needs of the mental health professional. Mental health practitioners have an ethical duty to provide responsible care, maximizing benefits and minimizing harm for their clients, and in order to provide effective care to their clients, practitioners must first be well themselves (Norcross & Guy, 2007). Accordingly, the regulatory associations of the major mental health disciplinary fields have placed responsibility for the care of the practitioner as a professional standard of practice (American Psychological Association [APA], 2017, American Counseling Association [ACA], 2014, and the National Association of Social Workers [NASW], 2021). Most recently, NASW used the specific terminology of "self-care" in their revised ethical code of standards. This renewed emphasis on professional self-care recognizes that proactive self-care reduces the likelihood of therapist impairment, enhances job satisfaction, and professional longevity (NASW, 2021).

## UNMET NEEDS

Lastly, if self-care needs are left unaddressed, therapists and their clients run the grave risk of health issues, a constricted life that lacks enjoyment from the everyday normative experiences of daily rituals or routines, social or family rituals, and family or community celebrations. There is ample evidence that untreated trauma has profound consequences that impact not only the individual but also families, communities, and society as well and has been identified as a public health concern (Substance Abuse and Mental Health Services Administration, 2014). Past traumas inform present-day health (Center for Substance Abuse Treatment, 2014) and significantly reduce quality of life, and diminish psychological and physical well-being. Finding ways to deeply understand the impact of trauma on self-care is of utmost importance for therapists so as to support their clients along the liminal experience of healing.

## CONCLUSION

This chapter explored the impact of trauma on self-care through the conceptual prism of liminality (Turner, 1967). Trauma presents as an amalgam of independent components that place individuals in a liminal time and space as they continue on their healing process. Part of the healing process involves self-care, which paradoxically pushes up against the fragmented "sense of self" that accompanies many trauma experiences. The complexity of traumas and multiple symptomatic responses can make it difficult for clients to engage in self-care practices as they move toward healing. Finding and utilizing a treatment approach, such as the ACT behavioral approach, may help clients take needed small steps as they engage in self-care practices.

Helping support clients to engage in self-care practices helps them build resiliency, which is a protective factor to mitigate trauma's effect (Beaumont et al., 2016). Over the long term, by building resilience through actions of self-care, the client can begin to reframe the experience of trauma into a narrative of deserving of care, compassion, and healing. Lastly, as trauma is ubiquitous and associated with a range of health care challenges, it affects all of us either directly or indirectly. As therapists train in supporting many clients in and across liminal spaces toward growth, it is imperative to understand the impact of trauma on self-care. Conceiving the "in-between" spaces of trauma and self-care as liminality experiences can be a critical conceptual framework for understanding, exploring, and appreciating the transitional times in which we all live.

# REFERENCES

American Counseling Association (2014). *2014 ACA code of ethics.* https://www.counseling.org/docs/default-source/ethics/2014-code-of-ethics.pdf

American Psychiatric Association (1980). *Diagnostic and statistical manual of mental disorders* (3rd ed.). American Psychiatric Association.

American Psychological Association (2017). *Ethical principles of psychologists and code of conduct* (2003, amended 2017). https://www.apa.org/ethics/code/

Baer, R. A., Lykins, E. L., & Peters, J. R. (2012). Mindfulness and self-compassion as predictors of psychological well-being in long-term meditators and matched non-meditators. *The Journal of Positive Psychology, 7,* 230–238. https://doi.org/10.1080/17439760.2012.674548

Baker, L. K., & Denyes, M. J. (2008). Predictors of self-care in adolescents with cystic fibrosis: A test of Orem's theories of self-care and self-care deficit. *Journal of Pediatric Nursing, 23*(1), 37–48. https://doi.org/10.1016/j.pedn.2007.07.008

Beaumont, E., Durkin, M., Hollins Martin, C. J., & Carson, J. (2016). Compassion for others, self-compassion, quality of life and mental well-being measures and their association with compassion fatigue and burnout in student midwives: A quantitative survey. *Midwifery, 34,* 239–244. https://doi.org/10.1016/j.midw.2015.11

Beech, N. (2011). Liminality and the practices of identity construction. *Human Relations, 64*(2), 285–302. https://doi.org/10.1177/0018726710371235

Bohart, A. C., & Tallman, K. (1996). The active client: Therapy as self- help. *Journal of Humanistic Psychology, 36*(3), 7–30. https://doi.org/10.1177/002210678960363002

Boyd, J. E., Lanius, R. A., & McKinnon, M. C. (2018). Mindfulness-based treatments for posttraumatic stress disorder: A review of the treatment literature and neurobiological evidence. *Journal of Psychiatry & Neuroscience, 43*(1), 7–25. https://doi.org/10.1503/jpn.170021

Briere, J. N., & Scott, C. (2006). *Principles of trauma therapy: A guide to symptoms, evaluation, and treatment.* Sage Publications, Inc.

Center for Substance Abuse Treatment (2014). Chapter 3, Understanding the impact of trauma. In *Trauma-informed care in behavioral health services,* Treatment improvement protocol (TIP) Series, No. 57. Substance Abuse and Mental Health Services Administration (US). https://www.ncbi.nlm.nih.gov/books/NBK207191/

Courtois, C. A., & Gold, S. N. (2009). The need for inclusion of psychological trauma in the professional curriculum: A call to action. *Psychological Trauma: Theory, Research, Practice, and Policy, 1*(1), 3–23. https://doi.org/10.1037/a0015224

Czarniawska, B., & Mazza, C. (2003). Consulting as a liminal space. *Human Relations, 56,* 267–290. https://doi.org/10.1177/0018726703056003612

Deblinger, E., Mannarino, A. P., Cohen, J. A., Runyon, M. K., & Steer, R. A. (2011). Trauma-focused cognitive behavioral therapy for children: Impact of the trauma narrative and treatment length. *Depression and Anxiety, 28*(1), 67–75. https://doi.org/10.1002/da.20744

Dindo, L., Van Liew, J. R., & Arch, J. J. (2017). Acceptance and commitment therapy: A transdiagnostic behavioral intervention for mental health and medical conditions. *Neurotherapeutics: The Journal of the American Society for Experimental NeuroTherapeutics, 14*(3), 546–553. https://doi.org/10.1007/s13311-017-0521-3

Dodgen-Magee, D. (2021). *Restart: Designing a healthy post-pandemic life.* Rowman & Littlefield.

Durkin, M., Beaumont, E., Hollins Martin, C. J., & Carson, J. (2016). A pilot study exploring the relationship between self-compassion, self-judgement, self-kindness, compassion, professional quality of life and wellbeing among UK community nurses. *Nurse Education Today, 46*, 109–114. https://doi.org/10.1016/j.nedt.2016.08.030

Foa, E. B., Hembree, E. A., & Rothbaum, B. O. (2007). *Prolonged exposure therapy for PTSD: Emotional processing of traumatic experiences: Therapist guide.* Oxford University Press. https://doi.org/10.1093/med:psych/9780195308501.001.0001

Franks, A., & Meteyard, J. (2007). Liminality: The transforming grace of in-between places. *Journal of Pastoral Care & Counseling, 61*(3), 215–222. https://doi.org/10.1177/154230500706100306

Frewen, P. A., Schroeter, M. L., Riva, G., Cipresso, P., Fairfield, B., Padulo, C., & Northoff, G. (2020). Neuroimaging the consciousness of self: Review and conceptual-methodological framework. *Neuroscience and Biobehavioral Reviews, 112*, 164–212. https://doi.org/10.1016/j.neubiorev.2020.01.023

van Gennep, A. (1908). *The rites of passage.* University of Chicago Press.

Goodyear-Brown, P. (2010). *Play therapy with traumatized children: A prescriptive approach.* Wiley.

Hayes, S. C., & Hofmann, S. G. (2021). "Third-wave" cognitive and behavioral therapies and the emergence of a process-based approach to intervention in psychiatry. *World Psychiatry, 20*(3), 363–375. https://doi.org/10.1002/wps.20884

Hayes, S. C., Strosahl, K. D., & Wilson, K. G. (2012). *Acceptance and commitment therapy: The process and practice of mindful change* (2nd ed.). Guilford Press.

Hayes, S. C., Ciarrochi, J., Hofmann, S. G., Chin, F., & Sahdra, B. (2022). Evolving an idionomic approach to processes of change: Towards a unified personalized science of human improvement. *Behaviour Research and Therapy, 156*, 104155. https://doi.org/10.1016/j.brat.2022.104155

Honkasalo, M. L. (2001). Vicissitudes of pain and suffering: Chronic pain and liminality. *Medical Anthropology, 19*(4), 319–353. https://doi.org/10.1080/01459740.2001.9966181

Jaarsma, T., Hill, L., Bayes-Genis, A., La Rocca, H. B., Castiello, T., Čelutkienė, J., Marques- Sule, E., Plymen, C. M., Piper, S. E., Riegel, B., Rutten, F. H., Ben Gal, T., Bauersachs, J. J., Coats, A. J. S., Chioncel, O., Lopatin, Y., Lund, L. H., Lainscak, M., Moura, B., Mullens, W., . . . Strömberg, A. (2021). Self-care of heart failure patients: Practical management recommendations from the Heart Failure Association of the European Society of Cardiology. *European Journal of Heart Failure, 23*(1), 157–174. https://doi.org/10.1002/ejhf.2008

Joinson, C. (1992). Coping with compassion fatigue. *Nursing, 22*(4), 116–122. PMID: 1570090

Jung, C. G. (1957/1960). The transcendent function. In H. Read, M. Fordham, & W. McGuire (Eds.), *The collected works of C. G. Jung* (Vol. 8, pp. 67–91). Princeton University. (Original work published in 1957)

King, A. P., Block, S. R., Sripada, R. K., Rauch, S. A., Porter, K. E., Favorite, T. K., Giardino, N., & Liberzon, I. (2016). A pilot study of mindfulness-based exposure therapy in OEF/OIF combat veterans with PTSD: Altered medial frontal cortex and amygdala responses in social-emotional processing. *Frontiers in Psychiatry, 7*, 154. https://doi.org/10.3389/fpsyt.2016.00154

Kissil, K., & Niño, A. (2017). Does the person-of-the-therapist training (POTT) promote self- care? Personal gains of MFT trainees following POTT: A retrospective thematic analysis. *Journal of Marital and Family Therapy, 43*(3), 526–536. https://doi.org/10.1111/jmft.12213

Kluetsch, R. C., Ros, T., Théberge, J., Frewen, P. A., Calhoun, V. D., Schmahl, C., Jetly, R., & Lanius, R. A. (2014). Plastic modulation of PTSD resting-state networks and subjective wellbeing by EEG neurofeedback. *Acta Psychiatrica Scandinavica, 130*(2), 123–136. https://doi.org/10.1111/acps.12229

van der Kolk, B. (2014). *The body keeps the score: Brain, mind, and body in the healing of trauma.* Viking.

Linehan, M. M. (1993). *Skills training manual for treating borderline personality disorder.* Guilford Press.

Mackay Yarnal, C. (2006). The Red Hat Society: Exploring the role of play, liminality, and communitas in older women's lives. *Journal of Women & Aging, 18*(3), 51–73. https://doi.org/10.1300/J074v18n03_05

Mannarino, A. P., & Cohen, J. A. (2017, September). *Trauma-focused cognitive behavioral therapy: What is it, how good is it, and why families need it.* http://www.societyforpsychotherapy.org/trauma-focused-cognitive-behavioral-therapy

Maté, G. (2022). *The myth of normal.* Avery Publishing.

McGuire, S., & Georges, J. (2003). Undocumentedness and liminality as health variables. *Advances in Nursing Science, 26*(3), 185–195. https://doi.org/10.1097/00012272-200307000-00004

Narasimhan, M., Allotey, P., & Hardon, A. (2019). Self-care interventions to advance health and wellbeing: A conceptual framework to inform normative guidance. *British Medical Journal, 365*, l1688. https://doi.org/10.1136/bmj.l1688

National Association of Social Workers (2021). *NASW code of ethics.* https://www.socialworkers.org/About/Ethics/Code-of-Ethics/Code-of-Ethics-English

National Technical Assistance Center for State Mental Health Planning, National Association of State Mental Health Program Directors (2004). *The damaging consequences of violence and trauma: Facts, discussion points, and recommendations for the behavioral health system* (pp. 1–136). https://www.nasmhpd.org/sites/default/files/Trauma%20Services%20doc%20FINAL-04.pdf

Nebrosky, R. J. (2003). A clinical model for the comprehensive treatment of trauma using an affect experiencing-attachment theory approach. In M. F. Solomon & D. J. Siegel (Eds.), *Healing trauma: Attachment, mind, body, and brain* (pp. 282–321). Norton.

Neff, K. D. (2012). The science of self-compassion. In C. Germer & R. Siegel (Eds.), *Compassion and wisdom in psychotherapy* (pp. 79–92). Guilford Press.

Norcross, J. C., & Guy, J. D. (2007). *Leaving it at the office: A guide to psychotherapist self-care.* Guilford Publishing.

Ohrnberger, J., Fichera, E., & Sutton, M. (2017). The relationship between physical and mental health: A mediation analysis. *Social Science & Medicine, 195*, 42–49. https://doi.org/10.1016/j.socscimed.2017.11.008

Shapiro, F., & Maxfield, L. (2002). Eye Movement Desensitization and Reprocessing (EMDR): Information processing in the treatment of trauma. *Journal of Clinical Psychology, 58*(8), 933–946. https://doi.org/10.1002/jclp.10068

Substance Abuse and Mental Health Services Administration (2014). *SAMHSA's concept of trauma and guidance for a trauma-informed approach*. HHS Publication No. (SMA) 14-4884.

Surtees, P., Wainwright, N. W., Luben, R. N., Wareham, N. J., Bingham, S. A., & Khaw, K. T. (2008). Psychological distress, major depressive disorder, and risk of stroke. *Neurology, 70*(10), 788–794. https://doi.org/10.1212/01.wnl.0000304109.18563.81

St. John, G. (2008). Victor Turner and contemporary cultural performance: An introduction. In G. St John (Ed.), *Victor Turner and contemporary cultural performance* (pp. 1–38). Berghann. https://doi.org/10.13140/2.1.3081.5523

Turner, V. (1967). *The forest of symbols: Aspects of Ndembu ritual*. Cornell University Press.

Van Dam, N. T., Sheppard, S. C., Forsyth, J. P., & Earleywine, M. (2011). Self-compassion is a better predictor than mindfulness of symptom severity and quality of life in mixed anxiety and depression. *Journal of Anxiety Disorders, 25*(1), 123–130. https://doi.org/10.1016/j.janxdis.2010.08.011

World Health Organization. (2014). *Self-care for health: A handbook for community health workers & volunteers*. http://apps.who.int/iris/handle

## CHAPTER FOUR

# Relational Trauma in the Family System

CLAIR MELLENTHIN and LEANNE ROHRBACH-STANGE

Research has shown that 90% of individuals within the United States will be exposed to at least one type of trauma event in their lifetime (Kilpatrick et al., 2013). As discussed throughout this book, traumatic experiences encompass exposure to and witnessing actual or threatened instances of death, serious injury, sexual violence, natural disasters, and other forms of vicarious traumatic events. Abusive experiences within family and home relationships constitute relational trauma and involve physical, emotional, sexual, and other psychologically harmful events (Russin & Stein, 2022). Relational trauma can have long-lasting consequences that reverberate throughout the family system, creating chaos and crisis within relationships and across systems. Children are particularly susceptible to relational and attachment trauma, as they are the least powerful members of the family system.

In her seminal work on childhood trauma, Lenore Terr (1990) describes the impact of trauma as "a sudden, unexpected, overwhelmingly intense emotional blow or series of blows that assaults the person from the outside" (p. 8). Families absorb these blows, and the impact on the relationships within the system and between members can be strained to a breaking point. Understanding how trauma impacts the family system and inherent relationships is crucial for the treating clinician, as is recognizing how to repair broken bonds, rebuild trust and security, and create a sense of safety within

*Trauma Impacts: The Repercussions of Individual and Collective Trauma*, First Edition.
Edited by Jessica Stone, Robert J. Grant, and Clair Mellenthin.
© 2024 John Wiley & Sons, Inc. Published 2024 by John Wiley & Sons, Inc.

the family relationship. Understanding the nature of the attachment system and how relational trauma disrupts optimal child development requires foundational knowledge of attachment theory.

## A BRIEF OVERVIEW OF ATTACHMENT THEORY

Attachment is one of the most comprehensively researched theories of human development (Cassidy & Shaver, 2016; Hughes, 2017). Bowlby (1988), who is often described as the father of attachment theory, described attachment as "an attempt to explain both attachment behavior, with its episodic appearance and disappearance, and also the enduring attachments that children and other individuals make to particular others" (p. 29). Attachment behaviors are the seeking out of others for comfort or security, and/or maintaining proximity to one who is "better able to cope with the world" (Bowlby, 1988, p. 27). Bowlby (1979) further described attachment behaviors as:

> any form of behaviour that results in a person attaining or retaining proximity to some other differentiated and preferred individual, who is usually conceived as stronger and/or wiser. Whilst especially evident during early childhood, attachment behaviour is held to characterize human beings from the cradle to the grave. It includes crying and calling, which elicit care, following and clinging, and also strong protest should the child be left alone. (p. 129)

Both children and adults engage in these behaviors when faced with fear, a sense of threat, loss, or abandonment. These behaviors are most observable when a person is experiencing fatigue, fear, loneliness, illness, or is overwhelmed by caregiving. The wide range of attachment behaviors that children can exhibit all have the goal of seeking connection and proximity to someone who can protect and care for them (Mellenthin, 2019).

The function of attachment is to create bonding and safety within and through relationships (Cassidy, 2016). A securely attached child and adult are more likely to modulate affect, express empathy, develop good reflective skills, and communicate emotional needs and wants in a reciprocal, attuned relationship. The parent or caregiver is able to meet their child's attachment needs in a consistent, predictable manner, helping to develop the child's internal working model of self (Bowlby, 1969). This core belief of *I am loved, loveable, and worthy of love,* helps the child develop healthy relationships with others throughout their lifetime.

In contemporary attachment theory, advances in neuropsychobiology have paved the way for understanding the importance of secure attachment throughout the lifespan. Porges (2022) describes how aspects of the social engagement system are functional at birth. This serves to enable infants and parents to co-regulate autonomic states via reciprocal cues of safety. This co-regulation provides the infant and parent with a neurophysiological platform from which attachment and the establishment of social bonds take place. Attachment and social bonds can be understood as "dependent on associations with feelings of safety" (Porges, 2022, p. 3).

Johnson (2019) describes these relationships with an attachment figure as a safe haven. This relationship to an attachment figure serves to "calm the nervous system and shape a physical and mental sense" and "where comfort and reassurance can be reliably obtained, and emotional balance can be restored and enhanced" (Johnson, 2019, p. 7). It is through these predictable patterns of connection that we can be assured that our everyday and existential fears are validated.

Attunement from these attachment figures from a young age "tunes the nervous system to be less sensitive to threat and creates expectations of a relatively safe and manageable world" (Johnson, 2019, p. 7). The formation of positive internal working models generates core beliefs about ourselves, others, and our communities that are internalized into a coherent sense of self. This sense of self is one representative of our inherent dignity, founded on mutual respect and love (Mellenthin, 2019). It is within this secure sense of self in attunement with our neuroception and interoception, that we are capable of having our needs met by an attachment figure. These repeated experiences continue to create positive models for those considered close to us in physical or emotional connection as sources of support (Johnson, 2019).

Felt safety over time provides security, as those close to us demonstrate not only accessibility but also accountability in their responsiveness. This security can be understood as a base from which we can begin to separate ourselves through the exploration of our surroundings with curiosity and conscientiously taking risks to develop competence and differentiate ourselves in the process. Johnson (2019) describes this "effective dependency" that this secure base provides as "a source of strength and resilience," which is responsible for the ability to internalize a "felt sense" of secure connection with others (p. 7). It is here, at this base, where we find refuge as we experience our attachment needs consistently met (Mellenthin, 2019).

A child is placed in a double bind when the person or adult most sought after for comfort is the one causing fear and terror in their life. Through these experiences, the child learns that their parent or caregiver is not only unreliable, but also frightening, and perhaps even violent. The parent lacks the ability to provide organized caregiving and may severely neglect or abuse the child (Mellenthin, 2019). In extreme situations, the parent(s) may fail to protect infants and children from danger, including physical and sexual abuse perpetrated by themselves or others, as they are unable to offer protection from their own negative affective states (Shapiro, 2010). Through these relationships, a child's internal working model of self develops into a belief structure of *I am not worthy of love or belonging. The world and others are unsafe, untrustworthy, and unpredictable* (Mellenthin, 2019). The internal working model that a child has internalized greatly impacts their ability to navigate the different phases of development and the ability to tolerate the changes and nuances of these years in an adaptive, healthy manner.

## HISTORICAL CONTEXT

Relational trauma has taken place in human relationships and family systems throughout history. However, until the 20th century, recognition of the trauma caused by relational violence and abuse in family relationships was not acknowledged. Freud was one of the first to observe and question the impact of relational trauma in his psychotherapy practice and initially declared that female hysteria occurred as a result of childhood trauma. He quickly retracted this statement and revised his premise that a woman's fantasy of sexual interaction was at the core of her debilitating symptoms. Prior to the acknowledgment and classification of Combat Neurosis in military veterans in the 1970s, family life and the secrets behind closed doors were social taboos and rarely talked about (Herman, 1992). It wasn't until the 1980s that the realization that many of the observable diagnosable behaviors that military veterans exhibited, which warranted a diagnosis of post-traumatic stress disorder (PTSD), also occurred in women and children who had experienced sexual assault and domestic violence (1992).

Prior to the late 20th century, women's and children's lives were shrouded in secrecy. In patriarchal societies, women and children were considered to be the property of men. In times of slavery, women and children could be bought and sold, separated without a thought as to the devastating impact this would have on them. Behind closed doors, there was no protection or refuge in violent homes. To speak about "the unspeakables" (Mellenthin, 2017) and the emotional, physical, and sexual violence that occurred within families was to invite shame, humiliation, and disbelief (Herman, 1992). Until the feminist movement of the 1970s, women and children in the United States were relegated to second-class citizenry. Women had no control over their income, finances, employment opportunities, and legal recourse. Currently, the Equal Rights Amendment (ERA) has still not been passed in the United States despite decades of advocacy.

Children have always been the most vulnerable to trauma, and until the last century, they were granted few protections (Courtney, 2020). Infanticide and beatings were viewed as acceptable parenting practices and continue even in modern times across cultures and family groups. Intimate partner violence (IPV) continues to be a scourge in our global community, as does children witnessing violence in their homes between caregivers, siblings against siblings, and with caregivers (Centers for Disease Control and Prevention [CDC], 2022b). There is currently no global understanding or standard on the impact of child abuse and IPV, even in modern times. In many areas of the world, child abuse and domestic violence are considered "a private family matter," and there are few protections granted.

Research has documented that children ages birth to three years have the highest rates of victimization (U.S. Department of Health & Human Services Administration for Children and Families Administration on Children, Youth and Families Children's Bureau [NCANDS], 2021). Children who witness domestic violence in their homes are 15 times more likely to be abused by their parents, including both the IPV perpetrator as well as the adult victim (Lieberman & Knorr, 2007). Relational trauma can have long-lasting consequences that reverberate throughout the family system. As noted elsewhere in this book, when children are exposed to multiple adverse childhood experiences (ACEs), the risk of psychological disorders increases significantly, as do rates of obesity, poverty, physical ailments, and disruptions to family life. It is estimated that 61% of adults in the United States experience at least one ACE before the age of 18, while one in six adults report four or more ACEs (Center for Disease Control and Prevention [CDC], 2022a). When children experience complex chronic trauma at the hands of those who are "supposed to be" the main people keeping them safe, this creates a painful paradox in terms of attachment. Even more devastating, what happens on a neurobiological basis in the face of unrelenting trauma creates lifelong difficulties and impairment in the child's brain, impacting mood, behavior, cognition, and emotions.

## PSYCHOLOGICAL IMPACT OF RELATIONAL TRAUMA ON THE FAMILY SYSTEM

Our literal understanding of the word trauma is founded in the Latin word for wound (Walsh, 2007). A wound is often a painful injury that breaks us open. Despite how the injury was inflicted, each of us heals differently from wounds, and relational trauma is no different. Even as members of a shared family system, our response to a potentially traumatic event may differ in psychological impact. Such impact is apparent in the relationship between caregivers of children within the family system, where the internalization of feelings experienced by the caregiver as a result of the traumatic event may lend to the externalization of behaviors in response to the child and their post-traumatic symptomatology. The Compound Effect introduced by Scheeringa and Zeanah (2001) more than two decades ago describes this impact in more detail.

## IMPACT ON NONOFFENDING CAREGIVERS

For nonoffending caregivers who have experienced secondary relational trauma within their family system, this impact is apparent in their cognitions and affect related to their own self, the child they care for, and the offender (Myrick & Green, 2013). This impact may be further complicated by the caregiver's thoughts and feelings toward the judicial system. Myrick and Green (2013) describe nonoffending parents of child abuse survivors as overwhelmed by emotional distress marked by feelings of guilt, as well as post-traumatic and grief symptomatology. These feelings of guilt are often internalized, manifesting in the form of "unrealistic standards, believing they should have had prescient knowledge that the perpetrator was dangerous" (Myrick & Green, 2013, p. 194). Situations in our daily living can also reinforce these feelings of guilt for caregivers, as the means of stability such as health, finances, housing, and employment may be affected. This demonstrates the ways how the experience of loss is often associated with traumatic events, demonstrating interconnectedness of trauma, loss, and grief, referred to as traumatic loss.

A caregiver may demonstrate feelings of guilt, denial, anger, and fear, among other feelings toward a child who has experienced relational trauma. They may respond with rejecting behaviors or overly apologetic responses, particularly if they were involved in the traumatic experience. Existing research (Coulter & Mooney, 2017; Fitzgerald et al., 2020; Myrick & Green, 2013) demonstrates that how the caregiver responds to their child impacts the child's mental health. It is in these moments following a traumatic experience when a child needs the protection of their caregiver the most, to provide felt safety and security to begin the process of repair and restoration after the trauma. When a caregiver cannot provide this, the child may experience forms of pain more significant than that of the initial traumatic event, as the attachment rupture deepens within the relationship. This is the result of a caregiver's inability to engage in regulatory functions, responsible for modulating a child's stress-response system. From a young age, a child is reliant on their caregiver to manage potential threats and associated stress (Scheeringa & Zeanah, 2001). Without the presence of a caregiver to co-regulate a potentially traumatic experience, children may demonstrate a triad of symptomatology, including "reexperiencing symptoms, numbing/avoidance symptoms, and hyperarousal symptoms" (Scheeringa & Zeanah, 2001, p. 801).

## THE COMPOUND EFFECT

Scheeringa and Zeanah (2001) have identified the interplay of attachment-seeking behaviors as the Compound Effect, in which the child and parent may be traumatized by the same or different events, but the effects of the symptomatology activate one another. When the child has experienced abuse at the hands of a perpetrator, they are directly affected by the traumatic event. The child's symptomology in response to the event may be indirectly affected by the caregiver's response to the event, which is informed by the caregiver's own post-traumatic symptomatology. Potential responses from the caregiver could include compromise in "reading the infant's cues, understanding their behavior, and responding to the child effectively" (Scheeringa & Zeanah, 2001, p. 809). In this same research study, Scheeringa and Zeanah (2001) detail three relational PTSD (RPTSD) patterns to describe the Compound Effect. These patterns are as follows:

1. Unresponsive or Unavailable
2. Overprotective or Constricting
3. Reenacting or Frightening

Much of these patterns are representative of the caregiver's own insecure attachment to the child, informed by their own experiences of relational trauma. The design of these patterns is repeated generation after generation in the form of intergenerational trauma until the attachment ruptures and wounds are healed.

## RELATIONAL POST-TRAUMATIC STRESS DISORDER PATTERNS

### Unresponsive or Unavailable Pattern

Caregivers who demonstrate Unresponsive or Unavailable patterns display "withdrawal symptoms" that can limit a caregiver's ability to read and respond, "sensitively to a young child who is similarly traumatized" (Scheeringa & Zeanah, 2001, p. 810). Much like in avoidant attachment, a cycle of avoid-approach attachment-seeking behaviors may develop. In this cycle, the caregiver, who is immersed in their lived experience, has little energy to engage with the child (Mellenthin, 2019). At times, this caregiver may be available or accessible, though this unpredictability has created a sense of insecurity for the child. In response, the child may display behaviors that move between rejection and neediness toward the caregiver. How the caregiver chooses to respond to the child perpetuates this cycle, as the caregiver may themselves engage in behaviors of rejection toward their child (Mellenthin, 2019). This cycle reinforces that love is painful to both the child and the caregiver. Because love is understood to be painful, the child and caregiver find their attachment requires deactivation to suppress hurtful thoughts, feelings, and behaviors associated with their relationship with others.

## OVERPROTECTIVE AND CONSTRICTING PATTERN

Behavior representative of the Overprotective and Constricting pattern indicates potential fear from a caregiver that their child may be traumatized another time. This pattern is also marked by feelings of guilt for caregivers related to their perceived ability to protect their child during the traumatic event (Scheeringa & Zeanah, 2001). Scheeringa and Zeanah (2001) concede that a caregiver's overprotectiveness "may occur independent of the child's exposure to trauma," although it could be a "possible response to traumatization" (p. 810). While this pattern may restore some feeling of control for the caregiver, associated behaviors may result in the formation of an insecure attachment between the caregiver and child, affecting the child's ability to develop "felt security or regulation of affect" due to the "limited opportunities for exploration and autonomy" offered by the caregiver (Mellenthin, 2019, p. 13). Through the traumatic event and the experiences that follow, the child is reminded that the world is a dangerous place.

## REENACTING OR FRIGHTENING PATTERN

Rather than displaying withdrawal symptoms representative of an avoidant response to a traumatic event, some caregivers will become flooded by intense emotions, trauma symptoms, and dysregulation. This flooding may bring about an "unwelcome preoccupation," where caregivers may continue to repeatedly ask the child questions about the traumatic event in such a way that may not only retraumatize the child but also frighten them (Scheeringa & Zeanah, 2001). These caregiver behaviors demonstrate a Reenacting or Frightening pattern of RPTSD. This pattern is similar to that of disorganized or chaotic attachment, where the child learns that their caregiver is not accountable or accessible to them. This child may engage in "attachment strategies that both seek out closeness and simultaneously avoid closeness when it is offered, resulting in a chaotic emotional existence" (Mellenthin, 2019, p. 15). Without the experience of a safe haven that a caregiver can provide, the child may be at increased risk of danger or further traumatization (Myrick & Green, 2013).

## FURTHER IMPACTS

These relational cycles within the family system can cause significant disruptions to the developing child, the quality of parental caregiving, and the escalation of emotional, physical, and sexual violence. The role of harsh parenting practices (physical aggression, hostility, the use of profanity, threats, withdrawal, and refusal to give affection) and partner-based trauma (physical, emotional, sexual, and psychological) within the home setting can have lifelong consequences for all family members (Fitzgerald et al., 2020). Afifi et al. (2017) found that harsh parenting is linked to long-term mental health effects, including lower self-esteem in children, suicide attempts, and substance abuse.

Research has demonstrated the systemic impact of relational trauma. Knapp et al. (2017) postulate that trauma increases negative relationship dynamics between adult couples, including more volatile conflict resolution styles. When this type of confrontation escalates to violence, children are often directly impacted—as direct targets, witnesses of violence against others, secondary victims of violence, and being injured while attempting to protect or stop the violence against their mother, in particular (Laing, 2000). This has a direct impact on children in the home who may respond with internalizing (symptoms of depression and anxiety) and externalizing (aggression, defiance, and hostility) behaviors that have a far-reaching impact on their social systems (Fitzgerald et al., 2020). This impacts the child's world by impairing academic functioning, peer relationships, struggles with authority figures, access to resources and social supports, and access to supportive adults. These adverse childhood struggles can then increase parental stress and conflict, creating a negative relationship cycle that escalates and permeates the family system.

Traumatic experiences and stressors can cause a host of ongoing problems, including access to support services and care. Lieberman and Knorr (2007) state, "family disruption, economic hardship, and relocation can further compromise a child's ability to rely on protective environmental supports to weather the developmental impact of traumatic stress" (p. 210). These further compound a child's developmental trajectory, as a child learns they cannot rely on their adult caregiver to offer protection from harm and violence. This may lead to a collapse in a child's ability to cope, regulate, and make sense of the world and relationships around them. The more repeated and pervasive the trauma occurs, the more likely the child will show "generalized and chronic disturbances in cognitive, social, and emotional functioning" (Lieberman & Knorr, 2007, p.210), features of disorganized attachment (Mellenthin, 2019), and the potential to continue the legacy of generational trauma in their own adult relationships (Fitzgerald, et al., 2020).

Research has further documented that increases in post-traumatic stress (PTS) and low levels of social support exacerbate the impact of trauma on the family system, causing heightened levels of stress, emotional volatility, reduced communication, and increased rates of separation and divorce (Coulter & Mooney, 2017). The upheaval and fragmentation of the family system and rupture with attachment figures can cause socioeconomic decline, low attendance in academic settings, mental health impairments, and involvement with the juvenile justice system, and are correlated with ongoing adverse experiences for all members of the family system (Williams, 2020).

## FUTURE RAMIFICATIONS (UNRESOLVED GENERATIONAL TRAUMA)

Research of intergenerational trauma began with the descendants of those who survived the Holocaust and Japanese Internment Camps of WWII (American Psychological Association [APA], n.d.). Since this time, the study of intergenerational trauma has been broadened to such atrocities as the removal of indigenous peoples, as well as violations of other historically marginalized populations (American Psychological Association [APA], n.d.). There are complicated losses associated with this form of trauma, which encompass forms of loss that may be difficult to assess or address (Walsh, 2007). The complications of such loss may be due to the quantity of losses sustained, as well as the qualitative effects associated with membership in historically disenfranchised populations. Intergenerational trauma is manifested across generations in numerous ways, such as suicidality, substance abuse, dissociation, and hypervigilance, in addition to "difficulty with relationships and attachment to others, difficulty in regulation aggression, and extreme reactivity to stress" (APA, n.d.; Fitzgerald et al., 2020). This symptomatology may appear different within the context of different cultures and societies. The transmission of this form of trauma is believed to be shared in parental communication about the event through interpersonal skills and behavior, in addition to shared attitudes and beliefs (APA, n.d.).

## INTERGENERATIONAL TRAUMA AND THE COMPOUND EFFECT

The circle of intergenerational trauma will remain unbroken when survivors cannot heal. Without the ability to heal, suffering may be perpetuated through acts of "self-destructive behavior or revenge toward others," inflicting harm to future generations by means of "cycles of mutual destruction" maintained by means of marginalization (Walsh, 2007, p. 210). In many ways, the RPTSD patterns that Scheeringa and Zeanah (2001) detail to describe the Compound

Effect depicts the inner workings of intergenerational trauma. Much of these patterns are representative of a caregiver's own post-traumatic symptomatology, which has been demonstrated to the caregiver by those who cared for them as a child. With the development of a negative internal working model about themselves, others, and the world, a series of beliefs and attitudes about safety and security is formed through parental communications. When these beliefs and attitudes are reinforced through these relationship exchanges, such patterns become even more valid to the caregiver and the child, making them more difficult to disprove. For a caregiver of a child who has experienced a potentially traumatic event, we can begin to disprove these patterns through the process of identifying what has been lost. This may be an intensive process for caregivers who have experienced intergenerational trauma, as it may become difficult to discern what forms of loss are their own rather than those of their families.

## CONTINUING BONDS TO HEAL

The practice of the Continuing Bonds model may allow a caregiver and child who have experienced loss due to a traumatic event consequent of intergenerational and relational trauma. The Continuing Bonds model describes how a caregiver can demonstrate secure attachment to who or what has been lost. Klass et al. (1996) first introduced the model within their edited work, *Continuing bonds: New Understanding of Grief.* Their work draws on the perspectives of 22 authors to create an emerging, shared consensus of the grief process. This model does not contend that there is a finality to the loss experienced but rather a change in the relationship. Such relationships can be reimagined into "spiritual connections, memories, deeds, and stories" to be shared across generations (Walsh, 2007, p. 210). This practice provides a caregiver and child the opportunity to make meaning of their trauma, "putting it in perspective and weaving the experience of loss and recovery into the fabric of individual and collective identity and life passage" in such a way that integrates rather than isolates them in their shared experiences (Walsh, 2007, p. 210).

## CONCLUSION

While humans can't escape exposure to trauma, interpersonal and intrapersonal trauma in family relationships creates systemic deleterious effects and impacts all members of the family unit, not just the primary victim and perpetrator. Without intervention and supportive networks of care, the long-lasting impact of family trauma ripples across generations. Families who experience relational trauma need access to support networks and resources, mental health treatment with a focus on the inherent attachment injuries and ruptures, and finally, a restructuring of the systemic interplays that can encompass safety.

## REFERENCES

Afifi, T. O., Ford, D., Gershoff, E. T., Merrick, M., Grogan-Kaylor, A., Ports, K. A., MacMillan, H. L., Holden, G. W., Taylor, C. A., Lee, S. J., & Peters, B. R. (2017). Spanking and adult mental health impairment: The case for the designation of spanking as an adverse childhood experience. *Child Abuse Neglect, 71,* 24–31.

American Psychological Association (n.d.). *Intergenerational trauma.* American Psychological Association. https://dictionary.apa.org/intergenerational-trauma

Bowlby, J. (1969). *Attachment and loss: Volume 1 attachment.* Basic Books.

Bowlby, J. (1979). *The making & breaking of affectional bonds.* Routledge.

Bowlby, J. (1988). *A secure base. Parent-child attachment and healthy human development.* Routledge.

Cassidy, J. (2016). The nature of a child's ties. In J. Cassidy & P. R. Shaver (Eds.), *Handbook of attachment* (3rd ed.). Guilford.

Cassidy, J., & Shaver, P. R. (2016). *Handbook of attachment* (3rd ed.). Guilford.

Centers for Disease Control and Prevention (2022a). *Fast facts: Preventing adverse childhood experiences.* https://www.cdc.gov/violenceprevention/aces/fastfact.html

Centers for Disease Control and Prevention (2022b). *Fast facts: Preventing intimate partner violence (IPV).* https://www.cdc.gov/violenceprevention/intimatepartnerviolence/fastfact.html

Coulter, S., & Mooney, S. (2017). Much more than PTSD: Mother's narratives of the impact of trauma on child survivors and their families. *Contemporary Family Therapy, 40,* 226–236.

Courtney, J. A. (2020). *Healing child and family trauma through expressive and play therapies.* W. W. Norton & Co.

Fitzgerald, M., London-Johnson, A., & Gallus, K. L. (2020). Intergenerational transmission of trauma and family systems theory: An empirical investigation. *Journal of Family Therapy, 42,* 406–424.

Herman, J. (1992). *Trauma and recovery: The aftermath of violence—From domestic abuse to political terror.* Basic Books.

Hughes, D. (2017). Dyadic developmental psychotherapy (DDP): An attachment-focused family treatment for developmental trauma. *Australian and New Zealand Journal of Family Therapy, 38,* 595–605.

Johnson, S. (2019). *Attachment theory in practice.* The Guilford Press.

Kilpatrick, D. G., Resnick, H. S., Milanak, M. E., Miller, M. W., Keyes, K. M., Knapp, A. E., Knapp, D. J., Brown, C. C., & Larsen, J. H. (2013). National estimates of exposure to traumatic events and PTSD prevalence using DSM-IV and DSM-5 Criteria. *Journal of Traumatic Stress, 26*(5), 537–547.

Klass, D., Silverman, P., & Nickman, S. (Eds.) (1996). *Continuing bonds: New understandings of grief.* Taylor & Francis Group.

Knapp, A. E., Knapp, D. J., Brown, C. C., & Larson, J. H. (2017). Conflict resolution styles as mediators of female child sexual abuse experience and heterosexual couple relationship satisfaction and stability in adulthood. *Journal of Child Sexual Abuse, 26,* 58–77.

Laing, L. (2000). Children, young people and domestic violence. In *Australian domestic and family violence clearinghouse issues paper 2*. Partnerships Against Domestic Violence, University of New South Wales.

Lieberman, A. F., & Knorr, K. (2007). The impact of trauma: A developmental framework for infancy and early childhood. *Pediatric Annals, 36*(4), 209–215.

Mellenthin, C. (2017). *Expressive arts in play therapy with teens.* [PowerPoint Presentation]. Wasatch Family Therapy.

Mellenthin, C. (2019). *Attachment centered play therapy.* Routledge.

Myrick, A. C., & Green, E. J. (2013). A play-based treatment paradigm for nonoffending caretakers: Evidence-informed secondary trauma treatment. *International Journal of Play Therapy, 22*(4), 193–206.

Porges, S. (2022). Polyvagal theory: A science of safety. *Frontiers of Integrated Neuroscience, 16*, 1–15.

Russin, S. E., & Stein, C. H. (2022). The aftermath of trauma and abuse and the impact on the family: A narrative literature review. *Trauma, Violence, & Abuse, 23*(4), 1288–1301.

Scheeringa, M. S., & Zeanah, C. H. (2001). A relational perspective on PTSD in early childhood. *Journal of Traumatic Stress, 14*(4), 799–815.

Shapiro, J. (2010). Attachment in the family context: Insights from development and clinical work. In S. Bennett & J. K. Nelson (Eds.), *Adult attachment in clinical social work*, Essential clinical social work series. Springer.

Walsh, F. (2007). Traumatic loss and major disasters: Strengthening family and community resilience. *Family Process, 26*(2), 207–227.

Terr, L. (1990). *Too scared to cry: Psychic trauma in childhood.* Basic Books.

U.S. Department of Health & Human Services Administration for Children and Families Administration on Children, Youth and Families Children's Bureau (NCANDS) (2021). Child maltreatment. https://www.acf.hhs.gov/cb/report/child-maltreatment-2021

Williams, A. (2020). Early childhood trauma impact on adolescent brain development, decision making abilities, and delinquent behaviors: Policy implications for juveniles tried in adult court systems. *Juvenile & Family Court Journal, 71*(1), 5–17.

## CHAPTER FIVE

# Trauma Impacts of COVID-19

JOHNNIE L. JENKINS, III

The traumatic impacts of the COVID-19 pandemic affected societal, cultural, and familial structures in profound ways. This modern pandemic compromised society's stability, leading to multiple family changes, such as different routines, work habits, and socialization patterns in an effort to comply with restrictions and health concerns. The COVID-19 pandemic created an environment of stress around the world, particularly due to the disordered unpredictable nature of the event.

Understanding the structures and frameworks of our society, culture, and system relationships, along with the impacts of an event such as a global pandemic, allows for emergence and healing. This chapter will present each concept for the reader, along with research to help illustrate known impacts to date, to assist in our conceptualizations of such impacts to the current and future generations. Best practices and policies that can assist in the recovery process will be presented, along with concerns and considerations for the future in terms of intergenerational and systemic repercussions.

## THE COVID-19 PANDEMIC

The COVID-19 pandemic unleashed a global health crisis with profound impacts on individuals, communities, societies, and systems. As the virus spreads rapidly across the globe, each country implemented measures such as lockdowns, social distancing, and mask mandates to mitigate its transmission.

*Trauma Impacts: The Repercussions of Individual and Collective Trauma*, First Edition.
Edited by Jessica Stone, Robert J. Grant, and Clair Mellenthin.
© 2024 John Wiley & Sons, Inc. Published 2024 by John Wiley & Sons, Inc.

These measures, while necessary, resulted in widespread and lasting disruption and trauma. The pandemic has caused immense physical, emotional, and psychological distress, leaving a lasting imprint on people's lives. The loss of loved ones, the fear of infection, the isolation from social connections, and economic hardships have created a perfect storm of traumatic experiences.

Individuals faced unprecedented levels of stress, anxiety, and grief during this time period. The trauma of the COVID-19 pandemic extends beyond the immediate health consequences, as it has exacerbated existing social inequalities and disparities, mental health needs, and has disproportionately affected marginalized communities. Frontline workers, including healthcare professionals and essential workers, have been particularly vulnerable to trauma due to their exposure to the virus and the immense pressure of their roles. We do not yet fully understand the long-term consequences of the pandemic on mental health and well-being, but it is clear that the collective trauma of this global crisis will leave an indelible mark on the society for years to come.

## STRUCTURAL AND FOUNDATIONAL CONCEPTS
### SOCIETY

The word "society" takes its meaning from a 15th-century French word *société*. The French word derives from the Latin *societas*, meaning "a friendly association with others" (New World Encyclopedia, n.d.). An important component within societies is that the associations within need structure to function. Sociologists define this social structure in terms of relationships, positions, actions, culture, power, and function (Calhoun et al., 1997). "Society is a system of usages and procedures, of authority and mutual aid, of many groupings and divisions, of controls of human behavior and of liberties" (MacIver & Page, 1949, p. 5).

People use a social context to view themselves in society. A social context is an environment framing interpersonal and individual behavior (American Psychological Association, n.d.). The context may include social and economic status, their cultural view of stressors, and if the context changed before and after the event. The context is the lens through which a person can understand themselves and the world around them.

### CULTURE

Falicov (1998; 1983) stated:

> Culture is those sets of shared worldviews, meanings, and adaptive behaviors derived from simultaneous membership and participation in a variety of contexts, such as language; rural, urban, suburban settings; race, ethnicity, and socioeconomic status; age, gender, religion, nationality; employment, education, and occupation; political ideology; stage of acculturation. (p. 14)

Society and culture remain consistent and change slowly under typical, noncrisis circumstances. When society and culture are stable, they show characteristics of homeostasis, predictability, and familiarity. People rely on these stable frameworks to navigate their daily lives, make decisions, engage, explore, grow, and strive toward a sense of belonging.

However, consistency and predictability are lost during crises, leading to rapid changes. Crises disrupt the established order, challenging the familiar and predictable patterns that people rely on. The sudden emergence of a global health crisis upends social norms, structures, and systems, and can prompt significant shifts in behaviors, attitudes, and functioning.

The need for rapid adaptation becomes paramount during a crisis. Society and culture undergo dynamic transformations as immediate challenges and uncertainties presented by the crisis are responded to. This period of upheaval can lead to the emergence of new social dynamics, the reevaluation of existing structures, and the creation of innovative solutions.

## Disruption

The COVID-19 pandemic disrupted our global society by removing predictability and causing stress and mental health problems. Stress, as described by Selye (1956), is the nonspecific sum of factors (activities, disease, drugs, etc.) acting on a body. It is imperative that we acknowledge and address how COVID-19 changed society, how individuals, families, and children respond to traumatic stress, and explore the best recovery practices for each.

Culture in society structures the worldview of people and shapes beliefs, norms, and values (Substance Abuse and Mental Health Services Administration [SAMSHA], 2014). The culture within a worldview can determine relationships between people, lives, and the overarching organization of the environment. Subgroups in culture "can be applied to describe the ways of life of groups formed based on age, profession, socioeconomic status, disability, sexual orientation, geographic location, membership in self-help support groups, on so forth" (Substance Abuse and Mental Health Services Administration [SAMSHA], 2014, p. 12). Culture is one of the foundational cornerstones of human life and disruptions permeate the entire system.

The COVID-19 pandemic made immediate societal changes. These changes included altered school routines, school closures, work schedules, work-at-home trends, resource shortages, and changes in retail shopping hours. Such changes influenced individuals, systems, and families, which ultimately changed relationships. Government-imposed lockdowns caused separation, social isolation, and educational impacts (Mathieu et al., 2020;

Meyerowitz-Katz et al., 2021). The lockdowns limited socialization, caused loneliness, isolation, and unhappiness in many people (Greyling et al., 2021), as well as damaged mental health (Kaubisch et al., 2022), and challenged relationships (Onyeaka et al., 2021).

## THE COLLECTIVE TRAUMA IMPACT OF COVID

The impact of COVID-19 on society and culture has been profound, leaving a trail of collective trauma (the psychological and emotional impact experienced by a group or society because of a shared traumatic event or series of events) in its wake. The pandemic has disrupted the fabric of our social connections, upended established routines, and exposed individuals and communities to prolonged periods of stress, fear, and uncertainty. The COVID-19 pandemic shattered the illusion of stability and predictability, thereby thrusting people into states of chronic trauma responses. The loss of loved ones, the overwhelming burden on healthcare systems, the economic hardships, and the isolation imposed by lockdowns have all contributed to a pervasive and global sense of collective trauma. The disruption of social networks, the erosion of fundamental trust, and the loss of communal rituals and gatherings have further deepened the trauma experienced by individuals and communities.

### *MENTAL HEALTH IMPACTS*

An increase in post-traumatic stress symptoms (PTSS), depression, anxiety, and attention-deficit hyperactivity disorder (ADHD) has been found as a result of people's experiences during the COVID-19 pandemic (Kaubisch et al., 2022). Studies have shown that mental health symptoms worsened as the pandemic continued (Pierce et al., 2021; World Health Organization [WHO], 2022).

> The COVID-19 pandemic has had a severe impact on the mental health and well-being of people around the world. While many individuals have adapted, others have experienced mental health problems, in some cases a consequence of COVID-19 infection. The pandemic also continues to impede access to mental health services and has raised concerns about increases in suicidal behavior. (World Health Organization [WHO], 2022, p. 1)

YoungMinds (2021) surveyed nearly 2500 youth ages 13–25 in the United Kingdom (UK) during the COVID-19 pandemic. The study asked if adolescents sought help during the pandemic to support their mental health. Of those surveyed, 75% felt the fourth lockdown was more challenging than previous ones. Additional results found that 67% thought the pandemic would have long-term effects on their mental health, yet 79% felt things would return to normal once restrictions ended. They reported:

1. 58% of respondents noted problems with loneliness and isolation
2. 51% of respondents had concerns about school/college/work
3. 39% struggled with frequent mental breakdowns
4. 36% had concerns about someone else getting sick
5. 20% worried about not getting mental health support
6. 19% stressed over family relationships
7. 14% did not know if they could get a job
8. 14% stressed when watching the news
9. 12% worried about their health
10. 12% worried about money
11. 10% worried about how they are portrayed in the media

Childhood traumatic experiences leave a ripple effect on children and their caregivers. During stressful, traumatic events, anxiety is a by-product. Children may feel uncertain about themselves, and their futures, and worry about their community and family.

Bridgland et al. (2021) surveyed 1040 participants from the United States (US), the UK, Canada, Australia, and New Zealand. The study measured emotional reactions, exposure to COVID-19, media exposure, post-traumatic stress disorder (PTSD) symptoms, disability screening, psychological functioning, depression, and anxiety. The results found that 13.2% were positive for PTSD. The researchers studied depression, anxiety, and stress using the Depression, Anxiety, and Stress Scale (DASS-21) (Ali et al., 2021). Results indicated that 47.3% of participants reported "normal" (not above average) levels of depression, 28.8% had mild–moderate depression, and 24% had severe to extreme depression. In the same study, researchers found that 15.9% of participants reported anxiety symptoms as mild–moderate and 14.5% of participants reported that their symptoms ranged from severe to extreme. The well-being of participants dropped in half by 55.9%. Psychosocially, adolescents surveyed reported significant distress in their interpersonal lives. Of those surveyed, 64.0% showed impairment, 62.8% had problems completing chores, and 27.6% had problems with training or education. The authors defined "impairment" as marked changes in performance and functioning, including changes in sleep patterns, eating, or mood. Additionally, Lawrence et al. (2022) also studied 530 responses from young people during the COVID-19 pandemic. Among these, 70% endorsed having mental illness or treatment. However, the scores indicated mild symptoms of anxiety, depression, and stress.

Bridgland et al. (2021) found that psychological criteria to measure PTSD did not accurately reflect what people experienced during the COVID-19 pandemic. In this study, researchers studied 1040 participants from 5 Western countries. They found that 13.2% met the criteria for PTSD on objective measures; however, their exposure was only to the lockdown. Lockdowns, the trauma event for their trauma criteria, are not an identified criterion for trauma exposure. Due to this, researchers discovered the participants had PTSD-like symptoms but did not meet the current criteria for a PTSD diagnosis. Their study found that those surveyed anticipated ($M = 8.98$, $SD = 5.24$) more negative events than they experienced ($M = 6.34$, $SD = 2.74$, $d = 0.49$). The YoungMinds survey also noted participant's misperceptions of their trauma experience. The classic definition of PTSD is exposure to an overwhelming event such as war, rape, or abuse (Schiraldi, 2009). The criteria for PTSD align in groupings of intentional human acts, unintentional human acts, and natural disasters, but lockdowns do not fit into these criteria.

## RECOVERY

This chapter has shown that the COVID-19 pandemic has impacted society's individual, familial, and systemic mental health, and exposed existing deficiencies in society's approach to trauma (Kazlauskas, 2017). Any specific models and approaches discussed in this section are recommendations to ease the issues imposed by COVID-19; however, they may apply to a number of traumatic events.

### *Adults*

The COVID-19 pandemic generated issues and influenced the recovery of adults. The pandemic spurred many stressors, which included the sudden and unexpected nature of the pandemic, financial hardships, increased parental burdens, and the fear of a loved one falling ill (Daks et al., 2022). Behar-Zusman et al. (2020) found that families confined to their homes during COVID experienced increased household stress, which increased the incidence of domestic violence (Drotning et al., 2022). Additionally, families had a decrease in household income, and they were twice as likely to have an increase in domestic violence during the pandemic.

Globally, adults experienced a 72% deterioration in mental health and a 78% increase in fatigue levels (Muldrew et al., 2022). Muldrew further found that one-third of people struggled with their caregiving roles, felt isolated, worried about the reduction in supply networks, stressed about a lack of information regarding the pandemic, stressed about their added challenges, and concerned about their well-being. Ramesh (2020) also discussed some global challenges in an interview with an executive at UNICEF, Naureen Naqui. The interviewer stated that globally, adults and families dealt with stigma; during the pandemic, discrimination occurred globally by healthcare workers, racial and ethnic groups, people with disabilities, and stigmatization of those who contracted COVID-19.

Other global trends during the pandemic included decreased healthcare coverage for refugees and displaced individuals, and it impacted learning spaces. Fifty-three percent of families had a decrease in their income (Pinkovetskaia, 2022), particularly single mothers (Taylor et al., 2022), and familial problems that existed prior to COVID worsened (Bailey & Jean-Pierre, 2020). Working from home, or remote work, also exacerbated these stressors (Tremblay & Mathieu, 2020, as cited in Charton et al., 2022).

## CHILDREN

Perry listed four suggestions to help children deal with trauma. The first suggestion is to promote public education about brain and child development. Initially, when the COVID-19 pandemic appeared, most public schools or worksites did not effectively inform the public and the children about potential traumatic exposures and their implications on the overall health. This caused confusion and a delayed reaction to the situation, ultimately eroding trust. The second suggestion is to respect the gifts of early childhood. Perry suggested that early intervention programs could assist children in meeting developmental milestones. Society does not currently incorporate these seamlessly into society. Early intervention programs can aid healthy development if trauma exposure occurs early. These programs should teach coping skills to address any existing traumas to lessen their effects. The third suggestion is to address the relationship deficiencies in society. Society's interventions during the COVID-19 pandemic resulted in many children experiencing stress and isolation. If children were lonely prior to the pandemic, isolation worsened this. Lastly, Perry suggests supporting families in healthy development. These societal changes need therapeutic techniques to heal children (2005).

Important therapeutic interventions and approaches are available to help children heal. One effective approach is to use trauma-based cognitive behavioural therapy (CBT) (Cavett & Drewes, 2012; Gil, 2006). These approaches allow children to share their experiences of the COVID-19 pandemic through narratives. These narratives provide children a place to tell the story about their experience in ways they can understand. Their words, stories, and creations allow them to share feelings associated with themes and symbols to describe their experiences. Since children do not always have accurate words to describe their subjective experiences, symbolic metaphors in play allow them to speak in ways they may not be able to verbalize.

The TraumaPlay™ model (Goodyear-Brown, 2019) also provides a valuable means for children to verbalize complex events such as trauma. The model allows a therapist to provide safety, assess the child's coping, soothe the child, improve the child's emotional literacy, expose the child to fears, help the child to understand their cognitions, look past the trauma, and regulate the child through the narrative.

The TraumaPlay model focuses on improving coping, soothing, and emotional literacy to reduce the need for defense mechanisms to avoid reality. The acknowledgment, accompanying mourning, and grieving stages align with the stages of a child's exposure to fear. A goal is to reach the last stage, or reconstruction. This is the stage where the therapist addresses cognitions, looks past the trauma, and uses self-regulation to produce productive trauma narratives (Goodyear-Brown, 2019).

Lee's (1970) four-stage trauma model (*impact, retreat, acknowledge,* and *reconstruction*) complements the TraumaPlay model. During the impact stage, individuals engage in depersonalization of the event. During the retreat, individuals are defensive and rely on defensive mechanisms to achieve homeostasis. These defense mechanisms may include depression, wishful thinking, fantasy, avoidance, suppression, and denial. During this retreat or depersonalization stage, children need therapists to provide safety and aid in reorganizing the traumatic memories. Issues are challenging to understand during the retreat or defense mechanism phase, so a client may create walls in an effort to block out the effects. The third stage, acknowledgment, shows individuals engaging in mourning or grief/loss from the event. The final stage is reconstruction within which individuals are encouraged to let go of past approaches and start with new approaches and a new view of themselves.

If children processed events of the COVID-19 pandemic using the Lee Model, this is how they may have used it in their response to the event: In the initial stages of the COVID-19 pandemic during the impact stage, children might have shown disconnection from themselves. They could have used depersonalization to cope with current uncertainties in the early days of lockdowns and isolation. When children realized that the COVID-19 pandemic was not temporary and would last longer than thought, they used defense mechanisms to cope. The retreat stage occurs out of a need to return to normal. Children could use fantasy, denial, or repression to escape the reality of the present situation. Children sometimes begin to realize they have lost family, friends, playtime, and events and mourn these during the acknowledgment stage. As the pandemic reaches its late stages, children reconstruct how they view themselves in the new era after the event. The reconstruction stage leads to the renewal of hope as things return to normal.

Children need many forms of support as they recover from the aftermath of the pandemic. Bartlett et al. (2020) listed recommendations to assist children in recovery. These recommendations include (a) knowing reactions to the pandemic may vary, (b) providing a sensitive and responsive caregiver, (c) understanding social distancing should not mean social isolation, (d) providing age-appropriate information, (e) creating a safe environment by practicing reassurance, routines, and regulation, (f) keeping children busy, (g) increasing a child's self-efficacy, (h) allowing caregivers to care for themselves, (i) seeking help if signs of trauma are present, and (j) emphasizing strengths, hope, and positivity.

During the pandemic, not every child responded the same way. Children and caregivers benefit from knowing that these differences are typical. Caregivers are central to a child's recovery and must remain healthy to help children. Caregivers should also empathize with children during a crisis. When therapists or caregivers communicate with children, they provide age-appropriate information. If the information is not developmentally appropriate, children will not have the tools to process it. If children experience a sense of safety, then they can progress through typical development scales. When children experience stressful events, one technique to use is to distract them and keep them busy. If parents keep to their routines, this helps children to gain self-efficacy. If trauma presents itself, seek treatment early and focus on strengths.

*FAMILIES*

Recovery from COVID-19 for families includes considerations from multiple areas: inequalities, mental health, familial dynamics, policy change, and changes within medical systems. Families inherently include impacted systems and these systems experience internal and external effects from many directions.

A byproduct of the pandemic was the highlighting of the need for societal policy changes. The recognition of flawed systems necessitates change and corrections. Lynch (2020) noted that policy changes should include universal health insurance, paid sick leave, wage insurance policies, tax reform, investments in parental leave, childcare, and education, and upgrades to government record systems. McCartan et al. (2021) suggested more investigation into the social determinants of health to address social inequities and poverty. To recover and prepare for the next pandemic, they further suggested investments in data collection sharing, more community-based care, providers understanding the lived experiences in services, improving interagency collaboration, investing in digital health records, and integrating physical and mental health.

It is particularly critical to consider addressing systemic racism and inequalities, and the need for long-term federal and state financial support (Bogan et al., 2022). Minority groups often experienced disproportionate negative consequences from COVID. One-third of Black families experienced three or more simultaneous economic or health-related hardships (Padilla & Thomson, 2021). In Black families, 45% lost jobs or had reduced hours compared to 31% of White workers (Swasey et al., 2020).

Grief counseling within families is another key consideration. Weinstock et al. (2021) noted that over one million children and adolescents lost loved ones to COVID. Their recovery depends on addressing the underlying grief, as individuals and within the familial systems. A lack of resources within the family and community resulted in numerous damaged relationships. The relationship damage occurred as schools and institutions closed, and a key element of recovery depends on government support of such community services (Weinstock et al., 2021).

These recommendations for recovery can address the instability many families faced during COVID. Highlighting inequities and difficulties within familial, medical, and governmental systems has the potential to lead to important change. Additionally, returning families to the routines they enjoyed pre-COVID, and the continuation of newly found priorities, will assist greatly as they strive toward healthy socialization patterns.

## Concerns and Considerations for the Future: Intergenerational and Systemic Repercussions

Although the rapid changes that occur during a traumatic event can be unsettling, they can also offer opportunities for growth, resilience, and hold the potential for a positive societal transformation. As demonstrated throughout the COVID-19 pandemic, crises can act as catalysts for innovation. These experiences can highlight the strengths and weaknesses of existing systems and inspire individuals and communities to adapt and develop new ways of functioning. These changes can shape the future trajectory of society and culture, leading to a new normal that reflects the lessons learned and the resilience gained during times of crisis.

As a result of these collective traumas, society and culture are undergoing, and will continue in the near future, profound transformations. The pandemic has forced us to reevaluate our values, priorities, and systems. It has sparked conversations about healthcare disparities (medical and mental health), economic inequalities, and the need for more resilient and inclusive societies. In the face of trauma, communities have come together. They have found strength and solace in solidarity and mutual support. The trauma of the COVID-19 pandemic is a catalyst for change, prompting us to question the status quo and seek new ways of living and relating to one another. It is through acknowledging and addressing the trauma that we have the opportunity to build a more compassionate, equitable, and resilient society for the future.

## CONCLUSION

The global COVID-19 pandemic produced a myriad of changes in society. Robinson et al. (2021) asserted that the pandemic deepened inequities and created new vulnerabilities. Isolation during the pandemic resulted in the loss of connections in existing communities and created new connections in new communities. Isolation changes the existing order in a society. A loss of order changes family relationships and as a result, some may feel powerless. This chapter introduced a number of the concerns faced during the COVID-19 pandemic for individuals, families, systems, and societies. Resilience, understanding, and support contribute to the recovery from such experiences; the emphasis on each has the intention of benefitting generations to come.

## REFERENCES

Ali, A. M., Alkhamees, A. A., Hori, H., Kim, Y., & Kunugi, H. (2021). The Depression Anxiety Stress Scale 21: Development and validation of the Depression Anxiety Stress Scale item in psychiatric patients and the general public for easier mental health measurement in a post COVID-19 world. *International Journal of Environmental Responsible Public Health, 18*(19), 10142.

American Psychological Association (n.d.). Social context. In *APA.com dictionary.* https://dictionary.apa.org/social-context

Bailey, J., & Jean-Pierre, J. (2020). The effects of COVID-19 prevention measures on families. *Child & Youth Services, 41*(3), 219–221. https://10.1080/0145935X.2020.1834915

Bartlett, J. D., Griffin, J., & Thompson, D. (2020, March 19). *Resources for supporting children's emotional well-being during the COVID-19 pandemic.* Child Trends. https://www.childtrends.org/publications/resources-for-supporting-childrens-emotional-well-being-during-the-covid-19-pandemic

Behar-Zusman, V., Chavez, J. V., & Gattamorta, K. (2020). Developing a measure of the impact of COVID-19 social distancing on household conflict and cohesion. *Family Process, 59*(3), 1045–1059. https://doi.org/10.1111/famp.12579

Bogan, E., Adams-Bass, V. N., Francis, L. A., Gaylord-Harden, N. K., Seaton, E. K., Scott, J. C., & Williams, J. L. (2022). Wearing a mask won't protect us from our history': The impact of COVID-19 on black children and families. *Social Policy Report, 35*(2), 1–33. https://doi.org/10.1002/sop2.23

Bridgland, V. M. E., Moeck, E. K., Green, D. M., Swain, T. L., Nayda, D. M., Matson, L. A., Hutchison, N. P., & Takarangi, M. K. T. (2021). Why the COVID-19 pandemic is a traumatic stressor. *PLOS ONE, 16*(1), 1–15. https://doi.org/10.1371/journal.pone.0240146

Calhoun, C., Light, D., & Keller, S. (1997). *Sociology* (7th ed.). McGraw-Hill.

Cavett, A. M., & Drewes, A. A. (2012). Play applications and trauma-specific components. In J. A. Cohen, A. P. Mannarino, & E. Deblinger (Eds.), *Trauma-focused CBT for children and adolescents: Treatment applications* (pp. 124–148). Guilford.

Charton, L., Labrecque, L., & Lévy, J. J. (2022). The COVID-19 pandemic: Global impacts on families. *Enfances Familles Générations, 40.* http://journals.openedition.org/efg/15277

Daks, J. S., Peltz, J. S., & Rogge, R. D. (2022). The impact of psychological flexibility on family dynamic amidst the COVID-19 pandemic: A longitudinal perspective. *Journal of Contextual Behavioral Science,* 97–113. https://doi.org/10.1016/j.jcbs.2022.08.011

Drotning, K. J., Doan, L., Sayer, L. C., Fish, J. N., & Rinderknecht, R. G. (2022). Not all homes are safe: Family violence following the onset of the covid-19 pandemic. *Journal of Family Violence,* 1–13. https://doi.org/10.1007/s10896-022-00372-y

Falicov, C. J. (1983). Introduction. In J. C. Hansen & C. J. Falicov (Eds.), *Cultural perspectives in family therapy* (pp. xiii–xix). Aspen.

Falicov, C. J. (1998). *Latino families in therapy: A guide to multicultural practice.* Guilford.

Gil, E. (2006). *Helping abused and traumatized children: Integrating directive and nondirective approaches.* Guilford.

Goodyear-Brown, P. (2019). *Trauma and play therapy: Helping children heal.* Routledge.

Greyling, T., Rossouw, S., & Adhikari, T. (2021). The good, the bad, and the ugly of lockdowns during COVID-19. *PLos ONE, 16*(1), e0245546. https://doi.org/10.1371/journal.pone.0245546

Kaubisch, L. T., Reck, C., von Tettenborn, A., & Woll, C. F. J. (2022). The COVID-19 pandemic as a traumatic event and the associated psychological impacts on families—A systematic review. *Journal of Affective Disorders, 319,* 27–39. https://doi.org/10.1016/j.jad.2022.08.109

Kazlauskas, E. (2017). Challenges for providing health care in traumatized populations: Barriers for PTSD treatments and the need for new developments. *Global Health Action, 10,* 1322399. https://doi.org/10.1080/16549716.2017.1322399

Lawrence, E. L., Jennings, N., Kioupi, V., Thompson, R., Diffey, J., & Vercammen, A. (2022, September). Psychological responses, mental health, and sense of agency for the dual challenges of climate change and the COVID-19 pandemic in young people in the UK: An online survey study. *Lancet Planet Health, 6,* e726–e738. https://www.thelancet.com/journals/lanplh/article/PIIS2542-5196(22)00172-3/fulltext

Lee, J. M. (1970). Emotional reactions to trauma. *Nursing Clinics of North America, 5*(4), 577–587.

Lynch, J. (2020). Health equity, social policy, and promoting recovery from COVID-19. *Journal of Health Politics, Policy & Law, 45*(6), 983–995. https://doi.org/10.1215/03616878-8641518

MacIver, R. M., & Page, C. H. (1949). *Society: An introductory analysis.* Rinehart and Company, Inc.

Mathieu, E., Ritchie, H., Rodés-Guirao, L., Appel, C., Giattino, C., Hasell, J., Macdonald, B., Dattani, S., Beltekian, D., Ortiz-Ospina, E., & Roser, M. (2020). *Coronavirus pandemic (COVID-19).* https://ourworldindata.org/coronavirus

Meyerowitz-Katz, G., Bhatt, S., Ratmann, O., Brauner, J.M., Flaxman, S., Mishra, S., Sharma, M., Mindermann, S., Bradley, V., Vollmer, M., Merone, L., &, Yemey, G.

(2021). Is the cure really worse than the disease? The health impacts of lockdowns during COVID-19. *BMJ Global Health*, 6, e006653. https://doi.org/10.1136/bmjgh-2021-005553

McCartan, C., Adell, T., Cameron, J., Davidson, G., Knifton, L., McDaid, S., & Mulholland, C. (2021). A scoping review of international policy responses to mental health recovery during the COVID-19 pandemic. *Health Research Policy and Systems*, *19*(1), 1–7. https://doi.org/10.1186/s12961-020-00652-3

Muldrew, D. H. L., Fee, A., & Coates, V. (2022). Impact of the COVID-19 pandemic on family carers in the community: A scoping review. *Health & Social Care in the Community*, *30*(4), 1275–1285. https://doi.org/10.1111/hsc.13677

New World Encyclopedia (n.d.). Society. In *New World zEncyclopedia.com*. https://www.newworldencyclopedia.org/entry/Society

Onyeaka, H., Anumudu, C. K., Al-Shafiry, Z. T., Egele-Godswill, E., & Mbaegbu, P. (2021). COVID-19 pandemic: A review of the global lockdown and its far-reaching effects. *Science Progress*, *104*(2). https://doi.org/10.1177/0036850421101985

Padilla, C. M., & Thomson, D. (2021, January 13). *More than one in four Latino and Black households with children are experiencing three or more hardships during COVID-19.* Child Trends. https://www.childtrends.org/publications/more-than-one-in-four-latino-and-black-households-withchildren-are-experiencing-three-or-more-hardships-during-covid-19

Perry, B. D. (2005). *Maltreatment and the developing child: How early childhood experience shapes child and culture* [Paper presentation]. Inaugural lecture: The margaret McCain lecture series. https://www.ifcc.on.ca

Pierce, M., McManus, S., Hope, H., Hotopf, M., Ford, T., Hatch, S. L., John, A., Konopantelis, E., Webb, R. T., Wessely, S., & Abel, K. M. (2021). Mental health responses to the COVID-19 pandemic: A latent class trajectory analysis using longitudinal UK data. *Lancet Psychiatry*, *8*(7), 610–619. https://doi.org/10.1016/S2215-0366(21)00151-6

Pinkovetskaia, I. (2022). Impact of Covid-19 pandemic on household income: Results of a survey of the economically active population. *Studia Universitatis Vasile Goldis Arad – Economics Series*, *32*(1), 43–57. https://doi.org/10.2478/sues-2022-0003

Ramesh, R. (2020). Building resilience and engaging communities to protect children and families during COVID-19 response and recovery. *Journal of Communication in Healthcare*, *13*(4), 256–259. https://doi.org/10.1080/17538068.2020.1843294

Robinson, L., Schulz, J., Ball, C., Chiaraluce, C., Dodel, M., Francis, J., Huang, K.-T., Johnson, E., Khilnani, A., Kleinmann, O., Kwon, K. H., McClain, N., Ng, Y. M. M., Pait, H., Ragnedda, M., Reisdorf, B. C., Rulu, M. L., da Silva, C. X., Trammel, J. M., Wiborg, Ø. N., & Williams, A. A. (2021). Cascading crises: Society in the age of COVID-19. *American Behavioral Scientist*, *65*(12), 1608–1622. https://doi.org/10.1177/00027642211003156

Selye, H. (1956). *The stress of life.* McGraw-Hill.

Schiraldi, G. R. (2009). *The posttraumatic stress disorder sourcebook: A guide to healing, recovery, and growth* (2nd ed.). McGraw-Hill.

Substance Abuse and Mental Health Services Administration [SAMHSA] (2014). *Improving cultural competence: A treatment improvement protocol* ([TIP] Series No. 59. HHS Publication No. [SMA] 14-4849). U.S. Department of Health and Human Services Substance Abuse and Mental Service Administration Center for Substance Abuse Treatment.

Swasey, C., Winter, E., & Sheyman, I. (2020, April 9). *Memo: The staggering economic impact of the coronavirus pandemic*. Data for Progress. https://filesforprogress.org/memos/thestaggering-economic-impact-coronavirus.pdf

Taylor, Z. E., Bailey, K., Herrera, F., Nair, N., & Adams, A. (2022). Strengths of the heart: Stressors, gratitude, and mental health in single mothers during the COVID-19 pandemic. *Journal of Family Psychology, 36*(3), 346–357. https://doi.org/10.1037/fam0000928

Weinstock, L., Dunda, D., Harrington, H., & Nelson, H. (2021). It's complicated—Adolescent grief in the time of Covid-19. *Frontiers in Psychiatry, 12*, 166. https://doi.org/10.3389/fpsyt.2021.638940

World Health Organization [WHO] (2022, March 2). *Mental health and COVID-19: Early evidence of the pandemic's impact: Scientific brief.* https://www.who.int/publications/i/item/WHO-2019-nCoV-Sci_Brief-Mental_health-2022.1

YoungMinds (2021). *Coronavirus: Impact on young people with mental health needs, Survey 4: February 2021.* Young minds UK. https://www.youngminds.org.uk/media/esifqn3z/youngminds-coronavirus-report-jan-2021.pdf

## CHAPTER SIX

# Suicide Risk and Social Isolation

JONATHAN B. SINGER and MARGARET ANN PAUUW

## DEFINITION AND OVERVIEW OF SUICIDE, TRAUMA, AND SOCIAL ISOLATION

### SUICIDE

Suicide is a leading cause of death among Americans (CDC, 2023). *Suicide* is defined as any death caused by injuring oneself with the intent to die. This means that the only deaths that are counted as suicide deaths are those where intent can be established, or if there is no other reasonable explanation. In 2021, 48,183 Americans died by suicide, with a rate of 14.1/100,000. The highest suicide rates (per 100,000) in the US are among white males (26.4), followed by American Indian/Alaska Native males (25), and Black males (14.1). While the largest number of suicide deaths is among adults, suicide is the third leading cause of death for 15- to 24-year-old Americans. Approximately, 6.5 million Americans are newly bereaved by suicide deaths each year (Cerel et al., 2019).

Although there are many suicide deaths, people are much more likely to know someone with suicidal ideation or attempt. In the US, it is estimated that 13 million Americans consider suicide every year (Ivey-Stephenson et al., 2022). *Suicidal ideation* is thoughts or feelings of suicide with or without intent to act. In 2021, approximately 22% of high school students reported thoughts of suicide (YRBS, 2023), and 4% of adults over 18 (Ivey-Stephenson et al., 2022). Suicidal ideation is different from *non-suicidal morbid ideation,* which is thoughts of death without suicidal or self-injurious content. *Suicide attempts* are any action taken with the intent of ending one's life, with or without injury. In 2021, approximately 10% of high school seniors reported a suicide attempt and 3% reported an attempt that needed medical attention (YRBS, 2023), compared with 0.6% of adults (Ivey-Stephenson et al., 2022). An *aborted suicide attempt* is where the person stops themselves, and an *interrupted suicide attempt* is where someone else stops a suicide attempt. *Non-suicidal self-injury* (NSSI) is the intentional immediate destruction of body tissue without the intent to die. While there is evidence that people who engage in frequent NSSI over a long period of time are also more likely to report suicidal thoughts (Whitlock et al., 2013), there is data to suggest that a subset of people use NSSI to reduce suicidal ideation (Herzog et al., 2022). People who have attempted suicide and lived are called *suicide attempt survivors*, and people who have lost a loved one die by suicide are called *suicide loss survivors*.

One of the most confusing aspects of suicidal thoughts and behaviors is that while connected, there is not a linear progression from thoughts to planning to action to death. People who are most likely to report thoughts and attempts are not the people most likely to die by suicide. As a result, the data presented in this chapter will sound at times contradictory. For example, although high school females were twice as likely to report thoughts of suicide and report an attempt (YRBS, 2023), high school-aged males were nearly three times as likely to die by suicide as high school-aged females (CDC, 2023). This gender paradox is explained in part because males use more lethal means than females, and that gender norms for males "produces a dual *concealing effect* (i.e., psychological pathologies packaged as gender identity/cultural practice), but in turn, a *delimiting effect* (i.e., limited expression and help-seeking)" (Oliffe et al., 2019, p. 316).

## TRAUMA

Because this entire book is about trauma, we will provide only a brief definition. Trauma can be the neurobiological, cognitive, and emotional response to one or more events that present a physical or psychological threat to oneself or others and generate a reaction of helplessness and fear (American Psychiatric Association, 2022). Trauma will be further discussed in this chapter as it intertwines with suicide and social isolation.

## SOCIAL ISOLATION

Social isolation is "an objective measure in which interpersonal contacts and relationships are quantitatively disrupted or non-existent" (de Jong Gierveld & Havens, 2004). Social isolation is typically assessed by considering the number of individuals with whom a person interacts in a given period, the frequency of social interactions, the number of qualitatively different types of relationships the person has, and the degree of intimacy involved in their interactions (Trout, 1980). Social connectedness is the objective complement to social isolation. Two key aspects of social isolation are social disconnectedness and perceived isolation (Cornwell & Waite, 2009). Social disconnectedness refers to a lack of social interactions and networks, while perceived isolation is an individual's thoughts and feelings about their social support, or lack thereof. The subjective experience of isolation is often referred to as loneliness. Someone can be socially isolated and not lonely, and someone can experience loneliness while having a large number of social contacts AND qualitatively strong social connections as in the cases of celebrity suicides such as Kate Spade or Anthony Bourdain (Singer, 2018). Researchers have looked at the relationship between social isolation and suicide risk in the following categories: marital status and living alone, social isolation, loneliness, alienation, and belongingness (Calati et al., 2019).

## HISTORY OF SUICIDE, TRAUMA, AND SOCIAL ISOLATION

Suicide has been part of recorded history for over 4,000 years. In 2100 BCE, an anonymous Egyptian took ink to papyrus and wrote a dialogue in which he tried to convince his soul to accompany him to the afterlife, offering the first known documentation and arguing in favor of the universal right to suicide (Evans & Farberow, 2003). Four thousand years later, on September 8, 2003, Garrett Lee Smith, the son of United States Senator Gordon Smith, an Eagle Scout, devout Mormon, and a college student who was struggling with substance use and depression, killed himself in his Utah apartment (Colburn, 2004). Although the definition of suicide as the intentional act of ending one's own life has remained consistent, the meaning of suicide has changed depending on the social and temporal context. The Egyptians died in a sociocultural environment that supported their choice of death and perhaps even honored it. Garrett Lee Smith died in a sociocultural environment that saw his suicide as possibly a sin, and definitely a tragedy of unfulfilled promise.

How did suicide move from being seen as a sin, to a medical illness, to our current conceptualization as a public health problem? During the early colonial period in the United States, suicide was considered a crime against both God and the state. By the 18th century, however, there were philosophical arguments challenging the moral prohibition against suicide. In 1777, philosopher David Hume even argued that suicide was a victimless crime that could potentially benefit society (Hume, 2010). Enlightenment-era beliefs about the order and rationality of nature inspired the first empirical investigation into suicide. In the late 19th century, Emile Durkheim analyzed suicide deaths in French towns and found that one of the major contributors to suicide was social isolation, which he described as a prolonged sense of not belonging and not being integrated into society (Durkheim, 1887). In the 19th century, the government took a more active role in organizing responses to social ills, creating a system of institutions that were intended to improve upon the community care that existed for centuries. Institutionalization had the unintended consequence of increasing isolation and social stigma associated with mental illness/suicidal thoughts and behaviors, and the intentional consequence of reinforcing the concept of "crazy" within those institutions (Estroff & Lamb, 1985; Goffman, 1961). By the 1960s, the combination of Kennedy's deinstitutionalization act, traumatized soldiers returning from the wars in Korea and Vietnam, and sociopolitical movements of the 1960s around racism, sexism, and homophobia, laid the groundwork for suicide to be recognized as a social problem (Minois, 1998).

The contemporary era of suicide prevention in the USA began with the 1997 congressional resolutions that recognized suicide "as a national problem and declares suicide prevention to be a national priority" (Garrett Lee Smith Memorial Act, 2004). Since then, there have been major advances in our understanding and recognition of the role of trauma and isolation in suicide risk, as well as efforts to provide community-based suicide prevention. Starting in 1998, the role of early childhood trauma in suicide risk over the lifespan was documented in a series of publications from the Adverse Childhood Experiences study (Dube et al., 2001; Felitti et al., 1998). In 2001, the USA published its first National Strategy for Suicide Prevention (U.S. Department of Health and Human Services, 2001). In 2004, Congress approved and allocated 84 million dollars for the Garrett Lee Smith Memorial Act for youth suicide prevention in K-12 schools, colleges and universities, and tribal nations, which resulted in reducing youth suicide by 79,000 youth over an 8-year period (Garraza et al., 2019). In 2005, Congress established and funded the first National Suicide Prevention Lifeline (converted to 988 in 2022). In 2007, Thomas Joiner proposed the Interpersonal Theory of Suicide (IPTS), which suggested that loneliness (as one of the key concepts in Thwarted Belonging) was one of three factors necessary for suicide (Joiner, 2007). This spurred a renaissance in theories, collectively referred to as ideation-to-action theories, that all recognized the role of loneliness in suicide risk (Klonsky et al., 2018). In 2015, Social Work established the Grand Challenge for Eliminating Social Isolation (Lubben et al., 2018).

## PSYCHOLOGICAL IMPACT OF TRAUMA AND SOCIAL ISOLATION

### Research

There is a complex relationship between social isolation and suicide risk, especially in the context of trauma. Humans have evolved over thousands of years to depend on social structures for survival. Social configurations not only influence behavior, but also genetics, hormones, and psychoneurological development (Cacioppo et al., 2011). Traumatic events change psychoneurological development, which can lead to mortality through physical health problems as well as cognitive, emotional, and psychiatric problems. People who have experienced trauma may self-isolate as a means of coping, even though social isolation has been linked with an increased risk of developing post-traumatic stress disorder and an increased risk of death from various causes, including smoking, obesity, cognitive decline, high blood pressure, and suicide (Cacioppo et al., 2011; Calati et al., 2019; Howick et al., 2019).

In contrast, social connectedness serves as a protective factor. People who are connected to others and have positive relationships are more likely to engage in behaviors that promote good health (Cacioppo et al., 2011). Beyond serving as a mechanism for survival, social support also promotes thriving, or the ability to make meaning of one's life, buffer oneself from adversity, and engage in activities that promote growth and fulfillment (Feeney & Collins, 2015).

### Personal, Familial, and Systemic

The relationship between social isolation, trauma, and suicide risk changes with the socio-developmental context, which itself varies across the lifespan. Data suggests that both social isolation and loneliness significantly increase suicide risk in youth. Early childhood neglect, a severe form of isolation and developmental trauma, contributed to a sevenfold increase in suicide deaths (Dube et al., 2001). Cohort studies have found that chronically high and increasing levels of loneliness early in life predict suicidal ideation in adolescence (Schinka et al., 2013). Among adolescents of all genders and across ethnoracial categories, social isolation predicted suicide attempts, while high levels of family and school connectedness and having a dense social network protected against suicide attempts (Boyd et al., 2022; Gulbas & Zayas, 2015; O'Gara et al., 2022; Whitlock et al., 2014).

As youth move from adolescence into adulthood, social connections shift from family and parents to peers and coworkers, and suicide risk changes by age and ethnoracial group. The suicide rate for college-aged adults is twice that of teenagers (CDC, 2023), and suicide rates are highest among same-aged young adults who never attended college (Schwartz, 2013). Of particular salience for adolescents and young adults, recent scholarship has found a correlation between youth who use social media to reduce social isolation-related anxiety and increased suicide risk (Scherr, 2022), and a positive correlation between decreased time on social media and decreased loneliness and depression (Hunt et al., 2018). As illustrated in Figure 6.1, suicide rates are consistently high among White adults (19 to 85+), increasing in the last years of life. Among Black and American Indian/Alaska Native adults, rates of suicide decrease with age. Among Asian and Pacific Islander adults, there is a bimodal distribution, with higher rates among 19 to 24-year-olds and 85+.

There is a well-established gender paradox by which men are 4 times as likely to die by suicide as women. In the USA, the suicide rates for the group with the most structural privilege, White men (32/100,000), are 10 times higher than for the group with the least structural privilege, Black women (3.3/100,000). The ITPS suggests that thwarted belonging (which is understood as loneliness and social disconnection), along with perceived burdensomeness and the capacity to die, are the three factors necessary for fatal or near-fatal suicide attempts (Joiner et al., 2021). Loneliness is one of the consequences of patriarchal norms that require men to conceal perceived weakness, discourage help-seeking, and sacrifice personal relationships for professional status.

Among older adults, social isolation contributes to poor health outcomes and increased mortality by limiting access to services and activities that are socially meaningful and health-promoting (Courtin & Knapp, 2017). Living alone,

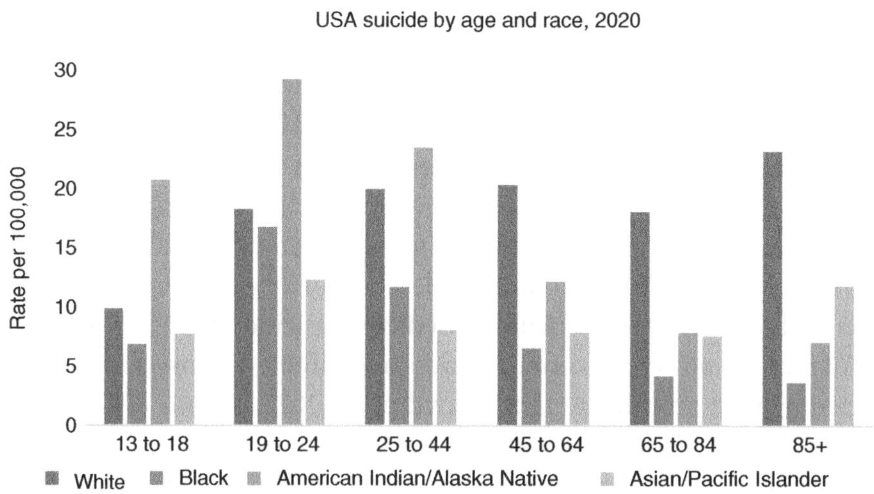



**Figure 6.1** USA Suicide by Age and Race, 2020. Note: Data were run by Jonathan Singer on March 4, 2023, using the WISQARS Fatal Injury site at https://wisqars.cdc.gov/. Source: Adapted from https://wisqars.cdc.gov/.

however, is not a proxy for social isolation in older adults. A meta-analysis found that among older adults, suicide ideation was strongly correlated with mistreatment, followed by perceived loneliness and poor perceived social support (Chang et al., 2017). Older adults who lived alone but who did not experience loneliness did not report increased suicide risk (Calati et al., 2019), compared to younger adults, for whom there is a stronger relationship between social isolation and loneliness. In earlier stages of the lifecycle, social connections are built into everyday interactions, whereas with older adults, social support generally requires more structure and planning.

## A 21ST CENTURY FOCUS; CONTEMPORARY ISSUES

As suicide risk has moved away from being seen as a sin, a medical problem, to a public health problem, both theories about and interventions for suicidal people have addressed social isolation. One of the few interventions that has been shown to reduce suicide risk in adults is a universal program for first and second graders called Good Behavior Game (Wilcox et al., 2008). One of the key elements of the Good Behavior Game is increasing student's connection to teachers, which contributes to a sense of connectedness to school and adults. Attachment-based family therapy for depressed and suicidal youth is a clinical intervention that repairs relational ruptures between youth and parents, increasing connectedness, and reducing loneliness and suicidal ideation in youth (Diamond et al., 2021).

Among adults, social isolation appears to be a greater risk factor for suicide in males than females. As noted above, the paradox of patriarchy increases social isolation in men by structurally disadvantaging experiences such as mental illness, ethnoracial, sexual, or gender minority status, financial disadvantage, and being single (Oliffe et al., 2019). A recent public health campaign, Man Therapy (MT), "attempts to change cultural norms to not only reduce suicide risk but also to reduce stigma about mental health, while encouraging men to view help-seeking as a sign of strength rather than weakness" (Frey et al., 2023, p. 139). Early evidence suggests that while the public health campaign did not reduce suicidal thoughts or behaviors in men, it did improve social support and motivation to get treatment (Frey et al., 2023).

The scholarship on social isolation, trauma, and suicide risk suggests that although there are structural barriers to overcome, the greatest challenge in the 21st century is to address the perceived disconnections and loneliness that accompany structural isolation. The early months of the COVID-19 pandemic created an experience of structural isolation that was unique in modern American history. The shelter-in-place orders prevented youth from engaging with same-age peers, adults from interacting with coworkers, and older adults from seeing family and friends. For those who lost loved ones during the initial quarantine and were unable to say goodbye was both traumatic and isolating. Losing a loved one from COVID-19 could be seen as a disenfranchised grief, as they were not able to practice cultural rituals, such as family gatherings and funerals. Recent research on suicide during the COVID-19 pandemic suggests a positive relationship between social isolation and loneliness and increased suicide risk (Blázquez-Fernández et al., 2023; Schnitzer et al., 2023).

One of the solutions to addressing social isolation is to expand our understanding of where mental health professionals and people can intersect beyond social service and healthcare settings. A useful frame is to think of our homes as first spaces, work and school as second spaces, and public community spaces such as cafés, parks, and libraries as third spaces (Bhabha, 2004). During the pandemic, we were confined to our first spaces. Then our schools and offices opened back up, though in a limited capacity. Third spaces are where people with the greatest risk for social isolation (older adults, people with serious and persistent mental illness) can be engaged, suggesting that they can be utilized as a protective factor against social isolation. For example, a third place could be a senior center where older adults go every day to see their friends and participate in activities. Libraries provide story time programming for children where young mothers connect with each other and build relationships. Expanding our understanding of social work services beyond the therapy office is essential to addressing social isolation in the 21st century.

## FUTURE RAMIFICATIONS IF UNTREATED/ UNADDRESSED WITHIN THE SYSTEM

In some ways, the relationship between suicide, trauma, and social isolation is complex. The reciprocal interaction of these three categories precludes simple intervention. When someone with suicidal thoughts or behaviors withdraws from others out of shame or embarrassment or removes themselves from socio-environmental contexts that could exacerbate their suicidal thoughts and behaviors (STB), they increase the social disconnection. In contrast, when someone is socially excluded or rejected, that can increase suicide risk. Trauma reactions can increase isolating behaviors and behaviors that others would reject (e.g., hypervigilance, impulsivity, and emotional lability). Because social isolation can serve as a risk and protective factor for suicide, it is unclear if increasing social connection will reduce or exacerbate suicide risk at the intersection of STB, trauma, and social isolation.

In other ways, however, the relationship between social isolation, trauma, and suicide is simple. Each is socially constructed and should be seen as a  modifiable aspect of contemporary society. As a society, we need to do a better job of building a world worth living in, reduce adverse childhood experiences and later traumas, and invest in social structures and social norms that increase social connectedness and reduce social isolation. At a micro level, this can look like reaching out to three friends every week and letting them know you are thinking about them. At a mezzo level, it can look like hiring social workers to work in third spaces such as libraries and public transit to provide services in the community. Third spaces such as parks, libraries, and community centers are often free public spaces, making specialized programming financially accessible for anyone to utilize. Because third spaces are outside of formal mental health services, they sidestep the shame and stigma associated with help-seeking and encourage natural supports to reduce social isolation.

If social isolation, trauma, and suicide risk are not addressed at a micro, mezzo, and macro level, it is possible we will continue to see traumatized youth grow into suicidal adults who see the world as a place not worth living in. "The great American promise is that we can be whatever we want to be. The great American tragedy is that most of our institutions—from schools to corporations—expect us to get there by sacrificing time with friends and family. . . The more time we spend with our loved ones, the easier it is to see when things are going wrong, connect them to people who can help, and help them build lives worth living" (Singer, 2018).

## REFERENCES

American Psychiatric Association (2022). *Diagnostic and statistical manual of mental disorders, text revision DSM-5-TR* (5th ed.). American Psychiatric Publishing Inc.

Bhabha, H. K. (2004). *The location of culture* (2nd ed.). Routledge.

Blázquez-Fernández, C., Lanza-León, P., & Cantarero-Prieto, D. (2023). A systematic review on suicide because of social isolation/and loneliness: Does COVID-19 make a difference? *Journal of Public Health*, fdad001. https://doi.org/10.1093/pubmed/fdad001

Boyd, D. T., Quinn, C. R., Jones, K. V., & Beer, O. W. J. (2022). Suicidal ideations and attempts within the family context: The role of parent support, bonding, and peer experiences with suicidal behaviors. *Journal of Racial and Ethnic Health Disparities*, 9(5), 1740–1749. https://doi.org/10.1007/s40615-021-01111-7

Cacioppo, J. T., Hawkley, L. C., Norman, G. J., & Berntson, G. G. (2011). Social isolation: Social isolation. *Annals of the New York Academy of Sciences*, 1231(1), 17–22. https://doi.org/10.1111/j.1749-6632.2011.06028.x

Calati, R., Ferrari, C., Brittner, M., Oasi, O., Olié, E., Carvalho, A. F., & Courtet, P. (2019). Suicidal thoughts and behaviors and social isolation: A narrative review of the literature. *Journal of Affective Disorders*, 245, 653–667. https://doi.org/10.1016/j.jad.2018.11.022

CDC (2023). *Fatality data, 2021*. National Center for Injury Prevention and Control, CDC. https://wisqars.cdc.gov/reports/

Cerel, J., Brown, M. M., Maple, M., Singleton, M., Venne, J., Moore, M., & Flaherty, C. (2019). How many people are exposed to suicide? Not six. *Suicide and Life-Threatening Behavior, 49*(2), 529–534. https://doi.org/10.1111/sltb.12450

Chang, Q., Chan, C. H., & Yip, P. S. F. (2017). A meta-analytic review on social relationships and suicidal ideation among older adults. *Social Science & Medicine, 191,* 65–76. https://doi.org/10.1016/j.socscimed.2017.09.003

Colburn, D. (2004, September 8). *Fraternity of sorrow.* The Oregonian.

Cornwell, E. Y., & Waite, L. J. (2009). Measuring social isolation among older adults using multiple indicators from the NSHAP study. *The Journals of Gerontology. Series B, Psychological Sciences and Social Sciences, 64B*(suppl-1), i38–i46. https://doi.org/10.1093/geronb/gbp037

Courtin, E., & Knapp, M. (2017). Social isolation, loneliness and health in old age: A scoping review. *Health & Social Care in the Community, 25*(3), 799–812. https://doi.org/10.1111/hsc.12311

Diamond, G. S., Diamond, G. M., & Levy, S. (2021). Attachment-based family therapy: Theory, clinical model, outcomes, and process research. *Journal of Affective Disorders, 294,* 286–295. https://doi.org/10.1016/j.jad.2021.07.005

Dube, S. R., Anda, R. F., Felitti, V. J., Chapman, D. P., Williamson, D. F., & Giles, W. H. (2001). Childhood abuse, household dysfunction, and the risk of attempted suicide throughout the life span: Findings from the Adverse Childhood Experiences Study. *JAMA, 286*(24), 3089–3096. https://doi.org/10.1001/jama.286.24.3089

Durkheim, E. (1887). In G. Simpson (Ed.), J. A. Spaulding, Trans.; Reissue edition *Suicide: A study in sociology.* Free Press.

Estroff, S. E., & Lamb, R. H. (1985). *Making it crazy: An ethnography of psychiatric clients in an american community.* University of California Press.

Evans, G., & Farberow, N. L. (2003). *The encyclopedia of suicide* (2nd ed.). Facts on File.

Feeney, B. C., & Collins, N. L. (2015). A new look at social support: A theoretical perspective on thriving through relationships. *Personality and Social Psychology Review, 19*(2), 113–147. https://doi.org/10.1177/1088868314544222

Felitti, V. J., Anda, R. F., Nordenberg, D., Williamson, D. F., Spitz, A. M., Edwards, V., Koss, M. P., & Marks, J. S. (1998). Relationship of childhood abuse and household dysfunction to many of the leading causes of death in adults: The Adverse Childhood Experiences (ACE) Study. *American Journal of Preventive Medicine, 14*(4), 245–258. https://doi.org/10.1016/S0749-3797(98)00017-8

Frey, J. J., Osteen, P. J., Sharpe, T. L., Mosby, A. O., Joiner, T., Ahmedani, B., Iwamoto, D., Nam, B., Spencer-Thomas, S., Ko, J., Ware, O. D., Imboden, R., Cornette, M. M., & Gilgoff, J. (2023). Effectiveness of man therapy to reduce suicidal ideation and depression among working-age men: A randomized controlled trial. *Suicide and Life-Threatening Behavior, 53*(1), 137–153. https://doi.org/10.1111/sltb.12932

Garraza, L. G., Kuiper, N., Goldston, D., McKeon, R., & Walrath, C. (2019). Long-term impact of the Garrett Lee Smith Youth Suicide Prevention Program on youth suicide mortality, 2006–2015. *Journal of Child Psychology and Psychiatry, 60*(10), 1142–1147. https://doi.org/10.1111/jcpp.13058

Garrett Lee Smith Memorial Act, Pub. L. No. 108–335, 42 U.S.C. 290aa, 290bb-34 and 290bb-36 (2004). https://www.govinfo.gov/app/details/PLAW-108publ355

Goffman, E. (1961). *Asylums: Essays on the social situation of mental patients and other inmates* (1st ed.). Anchor Books/Doubleday.

Gulbas, L. E., & Zayas, L. H. (2015). Examining the interplay among family, culture, and latina teen suicidal behavior. *Qualitative Health Research, 25*(5), 689–699. https://doi.org/10.1177/1049732314553598

Herzog, S., Choo, T.-H., Galfalvy, H., Mann, J. J., & Stanley, B. H. (2022). Effect of non-suicidal self-injury on suicidal ideation: Real-time monitoring study. *The British Journal of Psychiatry*, 1–3. https://doi.org/10.1192/bjp.2021.225

Howick, J., Kelly, P., & Kelly, M. (2019). Establishing a causal link between social relationships and health using the Bradford Hill Guidelines. *SSM - Population Health, 8*, 100402. https://doi.org/10.1016/j.ssmph.2019.100402

Hume, D. (2010). *Essays on suicide and the immortality of the soul*. Kessinger Publishing, LLC.

Hunt, M. G., Marx, R., Lipson, C., & Young, J. (2018). No more FOMO: Limiting social media decreases loneliness and depression. *Journal of Social and Clinical Psychology, 37*(10), 751–768. https://doi.org/10.1521/jscp.2018.37.10.751

Ivey-Stephenson, A. Z., Crosby, A. E., Hoenig, J. M., Gyawali, S., Park-Lee, E., & Hedden, S. L. (2022). Suicidal thoughts and behaviors among adults aged ≥18 years—United States, 2015–2019. *MMWR. Surveillance Summaries, 71*(1), 1–19. https://doi.org/10.15585/mmwr.ss7101a1

Joiner, T. E. (2007). *Why people die by suicide*. Harvard University Press.

Joiner, T. E., Jeon, M. E., Lieberman, A., Janakiraman, R., Duffy, M. E., Gai, A. R., & Dougherty, S. P. (2021). On prediction, refutation, and explanatory reach: A consideration of the Interpersonal Theory of Suicidal Behavior. *Preventive Medicine, 152*, 106453. https://doi.org/10.1016/j.ypmed.2021.106453

de Jong Gierveld, J., & Havens, B. (2004). Cross-national comparisons of social isolation and loneliness: Introduction and overview. *Canadian Journal on Aging, 23*(2), 109–113. https://doi.org/10.1353/cja.2004.0021

Klonsky, E. D., Saffer, B. Y., & Bryan, C. J. (2018). Ideation-to-action theories of suicide: A conceptual and empirical update. *Current Opinion in Psychology, 22*, 38–43. https://doi.org/10.1016/j.copsyc.2017.07.020

Lubben, J., Barth, R. P., Fong, R., Flynn, M., Sherraden, M., & Uehara, E. S. (2018). Grand challenges for social work and society. In R. Fong, J. Lubben, & R. P. Barth (Eds.), *Grand challenges for social work and society* (1st ed.). Oxford University Press.

Minois, M. G. (1998). *History of suicide: Voluntary death in western culture* (M. L. G. Cochrane, Trans. The Johns Hopkins University Press.

O'Gara, J. L., Gulbas, L. E., Suarez Bonilla, G., Manzo, G., Piña-Watson, B., & Zayas, L. H. (2022). Father–daughter relationships among Latina adolescents who attempted suicide: An exploratory dyadic analysis. *Family Process, 61*(2), 890–905. https://doi.org/10.1111/famp.12679

Oliffe, J. L., Broom, A., Popa, M., Jenkins, E. K., Rice, S. M., Ferlatte, O., & Rossnagel, E. (2019). Unpacking social isolation in men's suicidality. *Qualitative Health Research, 29*(3), 315–327. https://doi.org/10.1177/1049732318800003

Scherr, S. (2022). Social media, self-hjarm, and suicide. *Current Opinion in Psychology, 46*(101311), 1–6. https://doi.org/10.1016/j.copsyc.2022.101311

Schinka, K. C., van Dulmen, M. H. M., Mata, A. D., Bossarte, R., & Swahn, M. (2013). Psychosocial predictors and outcomes of loneliness trajectories from childhood to early adolescence. *Journal of Adolescence, 36*(6), 1251–1260. https://doi.org/10.1016/j.adolescence.2013.08.002

Schnitzer, P. G., Dykstra, H., & Collier, A. (2023). The COVID-19 pandemic and youth suicide: 2020–2021. *Pediatrics*, e2022058716. https://doi.org/10.1542/peds.2022-058716

Schwartz, A. J. (2013). Comparing the risk of suicide of college students with nonstudents. *Journal of College Student Psychotherapy, 27*(2), 120–137. https://doi.org/10.1080/87568225.2013.766108

Singer, J. B. (2018, June 12). We still don't fully understand suicide, but we do know what reduces it. *Fortune.* https://fortune.com/2018/06/12/suicide-prevention-anthony-bourdain-kate-spade/

Trout, D. L. (1980). The role of social isolation in suicide. *Suicide and Life-Threatening Behavior, 10*(1), 10–23. https://doi.org/10.1111/j.1943-278X.1980.tb00693.x

U.S. Department of Health and Human Services (2001). *National strategy for suicide prevention: Goals and objectives for action.* U.S. Department of Health and Human Services. http://www.ncbi.nlm.nih.gov/books/NBK44281/

Whitlock, J., Muehlenkamp, J. J., Eckenrode, J., Purington, A., Baral Abrams, G., Barreira, P., & Kress, V. (2013). Nonsuicidal self-injury as a gateway to suicide in young adults. *Journal of Adolescent Health, 52*(4), 486–492. https://doi.org/10.1016/j.jadohealth.2012.09.010

Whitlock, J., Wyman, P. A., & Moore, S. R. (2014). Connectedness and suicide prevention in adolescents: Pathways and implications. *Suicide and Life-Threatening Behavior, 44*, 246–272. https://doi.org/10.1111/sltb.12071

Wilcox, H. C., Kellam, S. G., Brown, C. H., Poduska, J., Ialongo, N. S., Wang, W., & Anthony, J. C. (2008). The impact of two universal randomized first- and second-grade classroom interventions on young adult suicide ideation and attempt. *Drug and Alcohol Dependence, 95*(Suppl 1), S60–S73. https://doi.org/10.1016/j.drugalcdep.2008.01.005

YRBS (2023). *Youth risk behavior survey: Data summary & trends report* (pp. 1–84). Centers for Disease Control and Prevention National Center for HIV, Viral Hepatitis, STD, and TB Prevention Division of Adolescent and School Health. https://www.cdc.gov/healthyyouth/data/yrbs/pdf/YRBS_Data-Summary-Trends_Report2023_508.pdf

# TRAUMA IMPACTS WITH SPECIFIC POPULATIONS

## CHAPTER SEVEN

# The Art of Being Brave: Building Resilience in Children with Medical Complexity

PATRICIA CAROLYN GILBAUGH

Resilience is not measured by what one has overcome. Rather, it is measured by the tenacity to keep overcoming. The most resilient children are those who overcome challenges and adversity repeatedly, with the full knowledge of the harm that will come to them. Many do this with courage befitting a superhero. An example of this occurs with chronically medically fragile children in the hospital setting. These children frequently know what they will face, including the multiple IVs, surgeries, recovery, and the pain they will go through as part of their medical care. This chapter focuses on the practical application of bravery—an art form of courage that children with medical complexity master at very young ages. These are the teachers of true resilience, and we have much to learn from their traumatic experiences.

*The art of being brave* describes the vulnerable population of children with medical complexity who are developing critical skills to manage their internal responses to the many external and internal stressors associated with their medical, neurological, and emotional conditions. The complex nature of being a child with medical complexity is formulated through the lens of repeated exposures to hospitalizations, doctors, medical tests, many procedures or interventions performed by licensed professionals, and caregiving requirements that exceed a typically developed healthy peer's requirements.

This chapter will explore medical trauma, extreme stress, resiliency, and how these manifest in young children. As part of this discussion, the authors will explore the trauma associated with chronic illness and surgery, including the medically necessary invasive procedures and the resulting perception of children who undergo painful procedures in a forced manner (i.e., being restrained or held down) performed by medical professionals. Specific focus will be on how repeated exposures to medical procedures can be mitigated or moderated by social conditions and caregiving skills. A case study is included to help with applying the concepts of building resilience in young children who require substantial support in being brave.

## CHILDREN WITH MEDICAL COMPLEXITY

Children with medical complexity (CMC) may have "a congenital or acquired multisystem disease, a severe neurologic condition with marked functional impairment, and/or technology dependence for activities of daily living," (Cohen et al., 2011, p. 529). Technology dependence involves the use of machines to support or sustain life (i.e., machines for breathing, mobility, or communication devices, or monitors and implants to continuously assess patient well-being). The physical and cognitive impairments contribute to the comorbid conditions of their mental, emotional, and social impairments. Often, children with medical complexity have needs that are not easily met by existing healthcare models. The silos of care the families must navigate are complex, and at times elusive. The balance between meeting physical or medical needs and meeting the needs of their mental health often leads families to weigh the exhausting costs and benefits of daily care.

All CMC share similar functional and resource-use consequences (Srivastava et al., 2005). These children and their families face constraints and financial strain due to functional technology devices, the high need for collaborative and coordinated care, expensive nutritional needs, and more. CMC require a high degree of medical oversight from their primary care physicians. These needs vary according to the intensity of their medical needs, their psychological and emotional needs, and the community's ability to support them (Cohen et al., 2011). The chronicity of their conditions typically involves multiple and lengthy hospital stays, a complex network of specialty care providers, and repeated surgeries and medical procedures.

Families of CMC face additional stress that research does not seem to capture. It is common to experience grief and loss of missed milestones, limited life opportunities, and the realization of intense deviation from typical childhood routines. Often, these children miss a lot of school, have very few close peer relationships, and miss out on life experiences that children typically have throughout their childhood. Experiences such as being invited to a friend's birthday party, attending a sleepover, or being asked to hang out after school are activities that CMC do not usually participate in. In examining daily life functions, assessment for typical peer socialization is a critical measure of potential protective factors, which enhance the building of resilience in children.

Moreover, little is known about the role of siblings and extended family in the lives and well-being of CMC. Practice experience suggests that siblings play a significant role in CMC and their ability to adapt to nontypical life activities. Siblings are frequently involved in helping with medical needs, such as assisting with feeding tubes or monitoring safety while parents attend to other family tasks. Extended family members can be a protective factor when offering support, and can also be a risk factor when engaging in feedback that is negative, judgmental, or condescending. Often extended family members who do not have close day-to-day contact with the CMC are superficial in their support or say things that have unintentional harmful consequences to the parents and/or child. For this reason, professionals should include in their assessment all the ways in which family members are helpful in terms of building resilience, and be open to learning about the ways these same family members can decrease the resilience in both CMC and their caregivers.

## MEASURES OF RESILIENCE IN CHILDREN

Garcia-Parra et al. (2021) defined resilience for children who have complex needs as:

> a reference framework for describing the positive aspects and mechanisms in an individual, group, material, or system that, when faced with a destabilizing and disruptive situation that threatens their integrity and stability, allows them to hold up, cope, recover, and emerge strengthened. (p. 1)

With this definition in mind, this section explores (a) the difficulty of how to measure resilience and (b) contemporary research that captures how resilience is developed in young people.

Kinard (1998) identified methodological issues in trying to define and measure resilience in children. Research over the past 25 years has resulted in little to no development in this area. What limited research that does exist, is limited to specialty populations and mostly about children in non-U.S. countries (Crowley et al., 2022; Pearce et al., 2015). A few studies have narrowed in on developing tools to measure resilience in adolescents (Nilsson et al., 2022; Pearce et al., 2015). Renbarger et al. (2020) conducted a meta-analysis of measuring resilience with the Child and Youth Resilience Measure (CYRM) tool. They examined the use of this evaluative tool across six countries. They found that while this research tool was invariant across age groups and genders, it had wide variances across communities. Social factors influenced the outcomes of the measures. This is not surprising, as it is common knowledge in the field of child development and child psychology, that resilience is often the product of layering protective factors and distinctive sources of stress.

Measuring resilience has been a long-time challenge, and it is particularly difficult to narrow the measurement criteria of children. What makes the difference between why one child is more resilient than another is baffling. Some children, even within the same family and social context, can adapt quickly and efficiently to major stressors better than another child. The characteristics of resilience as an understood psychological phenomenon have been difficult to understand in categorical terms. The existing research does not ask questions about perceived risk, trauma interpretation, or locus of control measures. A thorough examination of the literature revealed little to no research exists on measures of resilience for CMC.

Türk-Kurtçz and Kcatürk (2020) explored factors correlated with improving resilience in college students who experienced childhood trauma. They found that people who had higher traits of self-efficacy and an increased locus of control, experienced higher resilience. This finding is consistent with other research on the mitigating and moderating effects of protective factors discussed later in this chapter.

Based on therapeutic outpatient practice experience with CMC, measuring resilience within this subgroup of children needs more attention in two areas. First, the actual measures of what make a child more or less resilient need to be defined and developed for empirical purposes. Second, research is needed to clearly identify how children are able to overcome their medical experiences. Tools to measure resilience for this group should examine and include criteria that measure perceptions of risk-taking and a child's ability to analyze exposure to harm versus the pleasure of experiencing normalcy. Other measures should include interpretations of trauma and their ability to mitigate the effects of relational or relative traumas based on their actual experiences. For example, a needle poke can be traumatic for a child who is not used to this experience, but repeated exposures through the daily routine (i.e., a Type I diabetes diagnosis requires insulin shots) could diminish the perceived trauma and shift the narrative to routine life-sustaining adaptations. In addition, measures of resilience should include a perceptual analysis of how a child weighs the risks of harm against the ability to experience age-level milestones in child development. Finally, measures to acquire feelings of belonging to in-groups or "fitting in" with typically developed, non-CMC peers are an important factor in resiliency research with CMC. While caregiver resilience may indeed help mitigate the negative experiences children have, how children with medical complexity perceive their stress will greatly influence their ability to keep overcoming their adversity.

## THE IMPACT OF ACUTE STRESS

Researchers have defined Acute Stress (AS) as a summary of criteria defined in the Diagnostic and Statistical Manual 5th Edition (DSM5): a sudden and of short duration (less than a month) effect after experiencing a traumatic event (American Psychological Association [APA], 2013). The symptoms of AS include flashbacks, anxiety, avoidance, temper, sleep issues, attention issues, and depressive moods. AS in CMC is typically episodic but can evolve into a more constant state of hypervigilance, leading to post-traumatic stress disorder (PTSD).

Von Dawans et al. (2021) examined the current state of research addressing the impact of AS on the brain. They explored the biological aspects of how cortisol and other stress hormones produce physiological and biological responses. The complexity of psychological and cognitive effects of stress lacking in the studies of stress was also discussed. A general review of the literature to date reveals a lack of empirical research on the effect of stress on children and adolescents, although more research is becoming available as it relates to the effects of COVID-19 stressors. This type of research will be helpful in determining the impact of stress on children, but not specifically to those of children with complex or chronic medical needs.

Sandberg et al. (2000) looked at the effects of acute and chronic stress on the recurrence of asthma attacks. Not surprisingly, they found chronic stress had a significant likelihood of new and recurrent asthma attacks than single episodes of AS. This preliminary study might suggest that the chronicity of medical distress can play an important, and negative, role in a child's ability to cope with AS. It is unclear how resilience is affected by multiple episodes or the intensity of episodic AS. It is reasonable to conclude that accumulated episodic stress will eventually lead to symptoms of complex PTSD.

## MITIGATING TRAUMA FOR CMC

### Protective Factors

A need exists for conversations and research focused on mitigating and moderating factors for minimizing the potential harm for CMC due to the multiple medical procedures, stressful schedules, traumatizing events, and attachment disruptions. Among these factors, the roles of caregivers are given the most attention in the literature. How caregivers perceive the capabilities of their children is an area professionals are encouraged to become familiar with—as parents are typically the experts of their children. Being child-centered also means that professionals are parent-centered in their practice, as it relates to the layers of trust involved with treating CMC.

Rossen and Hull (2013) define protective factors as traits or characteristics that exist within a person or a person's environment that help mitigate the effects of trauma or stress. Mitigating the effects of trauma or stress includes navigating and reducing risk and fostering adaptive coping abilities to stress. Hulme (2018) identified typical protective factors, including nurturing and attachment, parenting and parental resilience, social connections, and social and emotional competence. The ability to self-regulate was included in the construct of emotional competence. As identified previously, CMC tend to be masters of courage. The ability of CMC to utilize self-regulation is a primary tool for building resilience and being brave.

Another area of protective factors includes spirituality and meditation. Research has shown spirituality to be a potential protective factor to mitigate emotional harm in stressful situations (Dey et al., 2021). Research has found spirituality to be a predictor for increased resilience and identified specifically as a factor to reduce the negative effects of stress on special needs children and their caregivers. Spirituality tends to provide a coping mechanism to provide hope for situations that are difficult to comprehend or explain. The sense of a higher power seems to provide supportive ideas about concepts related to finding purpose in suffering. While a review of the literature did not specifically reveal any studies that examined meditation for CMC, several studies point to meditation as having a significant effect on helping to reduce stress and increase resilience for children struggling with difficult situations (Jong et al., 2019; Patel et al., 2020; Stritter et al., 2021).

Hudson et al. (2014) described the single most protective factor for CMC as having at least one vigilant caregiver to ensure the child eats nutritious food, takes medications to prevent medical episodes, minimizes exposure to germs, and educates themselves about their child's diagnosis. Risk factors included stressors such as split custody and single-parent households. This is primarily due to the inconsistent and potential discontinuity of care for CMC. Homes that seemed to lack support and resources to fully support the complex medical care these children require can place CMC at greater risk due to the level of additional stressors involved (Hudson et al., 2014). Relationships with primary care physicians and available community resources were perceived as protective factors. A lack of these relationships was identified as a significant risk factor where these supports were either not available or there was a lack of resources to sustain them (Hudson et al., 2014).

## MODERATING FAMILY STRESSORS ASSOCIATED WITH CMC

Researchers examined the moderating effects of how children manage family stressors (Gaylord et al., 2003). These researchers identified that while age did not have a moderating effect on coping, gender does have a moderating effect on how family stress is managed and experienced. In this study, results showed that girls tend to decrease internalizing behavior as family stress increases, whereas boys' behavior as a result of increased stressors did not change. This finding indicates boys are at greater risk of not being able to cope or adapt when family stressors increase (Gaylord et al., 2003). An unintended finding from the research conducted by Tamir et al. (2022) suggests that girls between the ages of 8 and 10 with physical trauma are at a higher risk of developing PTSD. This finding is inconsistent with the findings of Gaylord et al. (2003) suggests that girls may internalize their stress-induced behaviors more so than boys, specifically within this age range, and expands on this notion to narrowing the scope of that internalization process as heightening during the development of prefrontal cortex.

Research has provided further evidence of gender differences in brain structure that are impacted by experiences with stress and trauma (Stepanous et al., 2023). Prefrontal cortex grey matter volume decreased in boys as their emotional distress increased, whereas the brains of girls were more impacted by socioeconomic stress (Stepanous et al., 2023). These differences may lead to variances in how boys and girls develop resilience or how they use protective factors to mitigate the effects of stress on their developing minds.

Raufelder et al. (2021) determined that youth who perceived social exclusion had a negative impact on the grey matter volume in the brain; however, perceived lack of social belonging did not. This finding has a considerable potential contribution to understanding how protective factors can buffer the impact of medical complexity on social, emotional, and cognitive development. Systemic change can influence resilience by building programs and services around the concepts of inclusion and decreasing the prominence of ableism. Since exclusion is a large part of decreasing resilience, developing programs around acceptance and inclusion of differently abled persons, including CMC, the stigma and problems that come from being classified as a person with disabilities will help guide the systemic changes needed for CMC.

## TRAUMA IN THE NAME OF MEDICINE

A thorough literature search resulted in no discovery of studies examining the effects of children being forced to submit to invasive and painful medical procedures without their consent or mental preparation. Often, these children are very young and preverbal and cannot provide informed consent on their own behalf. This is a stressful and traumatic experience for these children. In hospital settings, Child Life Specialists (CLS) are a trending expansion of medical care provided to children. The CLS assists children with self-regulating their emotional responses, as well as distracting them by using playful interventions to assist in ways they are affected by the recurring trauma. Medically induced trauma cannot always be avoided, such as in emergency situations; however, the needs of the young developing mind of CMC are being recognized in medical settings. Treatment providers are working to protect CMC from harmful exposure. This advancement is new and the need for research is vast.

## CASE EXAMPLE

Norah was born with a rare genetic disorder. Her parents learned during the fifth month of pregnancy that their baby had multiple congenital anomalies. The remainder of the pregnancy was considered high risk, and the baby's prognosis was grim, and unlikely to survive. Her parents were provided with options for medical interventions, including a late termination of the fetus. They chose to proceed with a natural outcome for the pregnancy, which ultimately resulted in a scheduled cesarean delivery of their baby.

At birth, Norah was not able to breathe on her own. She was immediately intubated and placed in the neonatal intensive care unit (NICU). Doctors examined her body and noted each of the physical anomalies. These included missing bones and organs, displaced organs, webbing of the feet and fingers, underdeveloped features of the body, hydrocephalus, spina bifida, a hole in her heart, and more. In summation, the totality of these conditions meant Norah would spend her entire life existing within the medical community—dependent on invasive medical procedures and medications to sustain her ability to stay alive.

Within the first 4 years of her life, Norah survived 21 major surgeries. These surgeries were mostly to repair the anomalies she was born with; however, some of these surgeries were intended to correct deficiencies in her ability to have certain functionality, such as restoring her ability to hear. Her lifetime of invasive surgeries, medical procedures, and medical visits resulted in accumulated complex and AS. At age 4, she underwent open-heart surgery in order to correct the structure of the arteries in her heart, and repair a hole in the atrial wall of the lower left chamber. The stress of this surgery, combined with the multiple previous surgeries and procedures, resulted in Norah developing symptoms of complex PTSD (c-PTSD).

Norah's symptoms included significant sleep disruption, including nightmares and night terrors. She experienced hypervigilance, especially regarding medical appointments, exaggerated startle responses to certain sounds and smells, and a generalized fear of being separated from her primary caregiver. Additional symptoms included an inability to maintain focus or complete tasks. Her cognitive function deteriorated, and her underdeveloped social skills regressed to clingy, dependent behaviors toward caregivers.

Due to her medical condition, Norah was unable to communicate her thoughts and emotions effectively. However, she was able to voice what she wanted to have happen to her. For example, when she was only 3 years old, she informed her doctor and nurses how she wanted them to perform a catheterization for a medical procedure. The self-advocacy was profound, and her mother recalled it as incredulous that a 3-year-old was able to exercise control over a procedure when the medical professionals initially wanted to hold her down. Rather, Norah was able to insist on not being held down and providing instructions on how to treat her respectfully, and with an ability for her to exhibit independence and courage so she could fully participate in a cooperative manner. This is a stark contrast to the multitude of previous procedures, including having IVs inserted, where nurses held her down and performed painful experiences against her will, and forced her compliance. The psychological trauma to both mother and child during these instances was pervasive and disturbing.

When Norah began play therapy, her presenting symptoms were consistent with both c-PTSD and periodic episodes of AS. Norah's progress was measured by her ability to express her worries, fears, and need for control through play behavior. She entered play therapy at age 6 and continued in therapy until adulthood. Even though the interventions shifted over time as she aged and developed, her trauma and need for control remained constant. The goals for therapy focused on helping Norah develop her internal locus of control and build resilience. This was taught using expressive language, self-regulation strategies, and the refinement of courage—developing a deep understanding at an age-appropriate level for what it means to be *brave*. By the time Norah was 18, she had experienced other nonmedical traumas. According to her mother, she was able to draw upon her experiences and resilience to transfer the skills associated with courage and autonomy to survive complex tragedy, including a sexual assault by a peer at age 13 and the suicidal death of her first serious boyfriend at age 14. Her complex healthcare needs somehow developed the intrinsic resilience she needed to survive insurmountable grief, loss, and victimization.

Norah learned through her therapeutic and life experiences that the act of being brave was an expressive art form in the sense that she relies on knowing she is her own best advocate and can selectively choose when to expose her vulnerability and when to mask it with strategies of self-regulation. She developed self-observation skills and uses the data she notices about herself to make decisions regarding compliance for undergoing procedures related to her healthcare. Over time, she has come to understand herself in ways that even mature, senior adults lack in depth and perception. This indicates that perhaps Maslow's concept of self-actualization is not necessarily about one's happiness and contentment, but rather about knowing one's limitations and ability to exhibit the appropriate amount of courage to mitigate traumatic duress. For Norah and many children like her, the *art of being brave* is the skill of building resilience, courage, and the tenacity to keep overcoming hard things in life.

## CONCLUSION

In summary, this chapter highlights the need for a clear definition of what resilience means and how can it be accurately measured for the purpose of social science research. Additionally, a better understanding of how trauma in CMC can be mitigated or moderated beyond the roles of caregivers and individual characteristics of child patients. Professionals working with this population are in need of better interventions, techniques, and strategies to facilitate better outcomes for CMC. Protecting the mental health of CMC involves giving these children autonomy over their bodies and trusting them to be in control of their lived experiences.

It is vital to look beyond evidence-based practice in this area and encourage professionals to examine practice-based evidence, and that building resilience in CMC involves teaching and demonstrating to the children themselves that they are capable beings and have the right and ability to be in control of their own bodies. This notion falls flat in the medical community; however, with the slow integration of using CLS, there is hope CMC will soon experience this type of support as a replacement for protocols such as being held down and forced to comply. Over time, this will lead to better outcomes and a reduction in stress and trauma symptoms.

The vastly diverse and unique population of CMC requires extensive knowledge about vulnerability, shame, and resilience. Professionals who work with this population do not necessarily need to acquire advanced learning about diseases, but rather focused learning about the effects of trauma on the development of CMC. Trauma-informed care necessitates a clear grasp of how to help children strengthen their ability to be more resilient in order for them to protect their mental health.

Complimentary alternative medicine is an area in which initial research suggests it could be very powerful in the healing of CMC and increasing their resilience. However, very little research is available that explores the impact of alternative medicines on CMC. Children need informed providers to work with them to help them feel in control of their bodies. CMC need supportive strategies and techniques, as well as moderating relationships (i.e., nurturing caregivers), in order to increase resilience—therefore, becoming braver.

The final thought to end this chapter is a resounding applause for the incredible acts of bravery performed by the youngest of minds and the frailest of bodies. To keep overcoming might be how resilience is defined, but the pokes and prods into tiny muscles remind us of the need to protect these special humans. We have much to learn from them, and they are such good teachers about life. Everything we need to know about being a good person is captured in the daily life of growing up in a hospital. The face of courage, the art of bravery—the concert of valor is the song of thriving and rising above.

## REFERENCES

American Psychiatric Association. (Ed.) (2013). *Diagnostic and statistical manual of mental disorders* (5th ed.). American Psychiatric Association.

Cohen, E., Kuo, D. Z., Agrawal, R., Berry, J. G., Bhagat, S. K., Simon, T. D., & Srivastava, R. (2011). Children with medical complexity: An emerging population for clinical and research initiatives. *Pediatrics, 127*(3), 529–538.

Crowley, T., van der Merwe, A. S., Esterhuizen, T., & Skinner, D. (2022). Resilience of adolescents living with HIV in the cape metropole of the western cape. *AIDS Care, 34*(9), 1103–1110.

von Dawans, B., Strojny, J., & Domes, G. (2021). The effects of acute stress and stress hormones on social cognition and behavior: Current state of research and future directions. *Neuroscience and Biobehavioral Reviews, 121,* 75–88. https://doi.org/10.1016/j.neubiorev.2020.11.026

Dey, N. E. Y., Amponsah, B., & Wiafe-Akenteng, C. B. (2021). Spirituality and subjective well-being of Ghanaian parents of children with special needs: The mediating role of resilience. *Journal of Health Psychology, 26*(9), 1377–1388.

Garcia-Parra, M., Negre, F., & Verger, S. (2021). Educational programs to build resilience in children, adolescents, or youth with disease or disability: A systematic review. *Education Sciences, 11,* 1–13.

Gaylord, N. K., Kitzmann, K. M., & Lockwood, R. L. (2003). Child characteristics as moderators of the association between family stress and children's internalizing, externalizing, and peer rejection. *Journal of Child and Family Studies, 12*(2), 201.

Hudson, S. M., Newman, S. D., Hester, W. H., Magwood, G. S., Mueller, M., & Laken, M. A. (2014). Factors influencing hospital admissions and emergency department visits among children with complex chronic conditions: A qualitative study of parents' and providers' perspectives. *Issues in Comprehensive Pediatric Nursing, 37*(1), 61–80.

Hulme, S. (2018). *Promoting a mental health wellness approach for toddlers in early childhood settings: Building resilience through the development of protective factors (Publication No. 10750788)*. [Dissertation]. Oakland University. ProQuest Dissertations and Theses Global.

Jong, M. C., Boers, I., van Wietmarschen, H. A., Tromp, E., Busari, J. O., Wennekes, R., Snoeck, I., Bekhof, J., & Vlieger, A. M. (2019). Hypnotherapy or transcendental meditation versus progressive muscle relaxation exercises in the treatment of children with primary headaches: A multi-centre, pragmatic, randomised clinical study. *European Journal of Pediatrics, 178*(2), 147–154.

Kinard, E. M. (1998). Methodological issues in assessing resilience in maltreated children. *Child Abuse & Neglect, 22*(7), 669–680.

Nilsson, D., Svedin, C. G., Hall, F., Kazemi, E., & Dahlstrom, O. (2022). Psychometric properties of the Adolescent Resilience Questionnaire (ARQ) in a sample of Swedish adolescents. *BMC Psychiatry, 22*(1), 1–12.

Patel, H., Nguyen, K. H., Lehman, E., Mainali, G., Duda, L., Byler, D., & Kumar, A. (2020). Use of complementary and alternative medicine in children with Tourette syndrome. *Journal of Child Neurology, 35*(8), 512–516. https://doi.org/10.1177/0883073820913670

Pearce, M. E., Jongbloed, K. A., Richardson, C. G., Henderson, E. W., Pooyak, S. D., Oviedo-Joekes, E., Christian, W. M., Schechter, M. T., Spittal, P. M., & Cedar Project Partnership (2015). The Cedar Project: Resilience in the face of HIV vulnerability within a cohort study involving young Indigenous people who use drugs in three Canadian cities. *BMC Public Health, 15*(1), 1–12.

Raufelder, D., Neumann, N., Domin, M., Lorenz, R. C., Gleich, T., Golde, S., Romund, L., Beck, A., & Horferichter, F. (2021). Do belonging and social exclusion at school affect structural brain development during adolescence? *Child Development, 92*(6), 2213–2223.

Renbarger, R. L., Padgett, R. N., Cowden, R. G., Govender, K., Yilmaz, M. Z., Scott, L. M., Makhnack, A. V., Novotny, J. S., Nugent, G., Rosenbaum, L., & Kremenkova, L. (2020). Culturally relevant resilience: A psychometric meta-analysis of the Child and Youth Resilience Measure (CYRM). *Journal of Research on Adolescence (Wiley-Blackwell), 30*(4), 896–912.

Rossen, E., & Hull, R. (Eds.) (2013). *Supporting and educating traumatized students: A guide for school-based professionals*. Oxford University Press.

Sandberg, S., Patton, J. Y., Ahola, S., McCann, D. C., McGuinness, D., Hillary, C. R., & Oja, H. (2000). The role of acute and chronic stress in asthma attacks in children. *Lancet, 356*(2934), 982.

Srivastava, R., Stone, B. L., & Murphy, N. A. (2005). Hospitalist care of the medically complex child. *Pediatric Clinics of North America, 52*(4), 1165–1187.

Stepanous, J., Munford, L., Qualter, P., Banaschewski, T., Needs, F., & Elliott, R. (2023). Social environment and brain structure in adolescent mental health: A cross-sectional structural equation modeling study using IMAGEN data. *PLoS One, 17*(1), 1–24.

Stritter, W., Everding, J., Luchte, J., Eggert, A., & Seifert, G. (2021). Yoga, meditation and mindfulness in pediatric oncology—A review of literature. *Complementary Therapies in Medicine, 63*. https://doi.org/10.1016/j.ctim.2021.102791

Tamir, T. T., Kassa, S. F., & Gebeyehu, D. A. (2022). A multi-institutional study of post-traumatic stress disorder and its risk factors in Ethiopian pediatric patients with physical trauma. *BMC Psychiatry, 22*(1), 1–9.

Türk-Kurtçz, T., & Kcatürk, M. (2020). The role of childhood traumas, emotional self-efficacy, and internal-external locus of control in predicting psychological resilience. *International Journal of Education and Literacy Studies, 8*(3), 105–115.

## CHAPTER EIGHT

# Disasters

STEVEN L. BISTRICKY, ZARA KENIGSBERG, MAURICIO MONTES, ALEXA RIOBUENO-NAYLOR, and BETTY S. LAI

## DEFINITION AND OVERVIEW

Disasters are large-scale, potentially traumatic events (Furr et al., 2010). Disasters not only include extreme events such as earthquakes, hurricanes, and floods, but also biological pandemics or terrorist events such as the 2013 Boston Marathon bombing and the 2022 Colorado Springs Club Q mass shooting. Largely due to climate change, climate-impacted disasters such as hurricanes are increasing in frequency and intensity (Ornes, 2018). Between 2017 and 2019, the United States experienced 44 disasters that caused over 1 billion dollars in damages (Smith, 2020). Experts estimate that Generation Alpha, those born between 2010 and 2025, will experience two-to-seven-times as many disaster events as their grandparents (Thiery et al., 2021). In this chapter, we review evidence from psychology and disaster sciences, focusing on how disasters impact mental health and how risk factors and protective factors can influence the degree of impact. We also provide a case example and discuss future directions for the field.

## PSYCHOLOGICAL IMPACTS OF DISASTERS

Although resilience, or the ability to "bounce forward" and adapt (Mayena et al., 2011), is the most common reaction after disaster exposure (Galatzer-Levy et al., 2018; Lai et al., 2021; Lowe et al., 2021), many individuals develop

*Trauma Impacts: The Repercussions of Individual and Collective Trauma*, First Edition.
Edited by Jessica Stone, Robert J. Grant, and Clair Mellenthin.
© 2024 John Wiley & Sons, Inc. Published 2024 by John Wiley & Sons, Inc.

symptoms of mental health distress (Lee et al., 2020; Neria et al., 2008). For example, a systematic review examining the psychological impact of disasters and pandemics in geographically diverse child and adult samples found that six months post-disaster, 28% of individuals developed clinically significant depressive symptoms, 23% developed anxiety symptoms, and 24% developed post-traumatic stress (PTS) symptoms (Newnham et al., 2022).

PTS symptoms include recurring, involuntary, and intrusive memories of the disaster; avoidance of reminders of disaster; negative alterations in thinking and mood; and greater arousal and reactivity (American Psychiatric Association [APA], 2022). Common post-disaster psychological responses also include internalizing (e.g., depression and anxiety; Lowe et al., 2019) and externalizing difficulties (e.g., aggression and disruptive behavior; Self-Brown et al., 2017). Post-traumatic psychiatric symptoms are often comorbid and chronic within individuals (Qassem et al., 2021). For example, comorbid symptoms of PTS and depression have been reported as far as 15 months post-disaster, contributing to greater symptom severity and a prolonged course of symptoms (Lai et al., 2013).

Cultural conceptions shape how people understand post-disaster psychological symptoms. For instance, *ataques de nervios* ("attack of the nerves") describes a Latine cultural concept of distress (Baggerly et al., 2022; Rahmani et al., 2022). Symptoms include intense anxiety, loss of control, rage, aggressiveness, amnesia, depersonalization, and derealization (Alcántara & Lewis-Fernández, 2016; APA, 2022). By the same token, individuals' core assumptions and beliefs about the world, themselves, and others can be disrupted in the aftermath of a disaster (García et al., 2015). As survivors process the impact of the disaster and new realities of life, they may develop meaning from the event and experience positive change, such as improvements in relationships, increased spiritual well-being, a greater appreciation of life, and the identification of new possibilities and priorities (Tedeschi et al., 2018). This *post-traumatic growth* does not negate the experience of symptoms and distress and may in fact be developed from processing those experiences.

## RISK FACTORS FOR PSYCHOLOGICAL IMPACTS OF DISASTERS

Disasters do not affect all communities equally. Communities have varying degrees of *social vulnerability*, which refers to the susceptibility of communities to the adverse consequences of disasters, due to factors such as limited access to resources. Socially vulnerable communities endure greater disaster-related loss and exert more effort to protect their resources when a disaster occurs. In disaster contexts, low-income communities, ethnically and racially marginalized groups, and children and older adults tend to experience the most social vulnerability (Benevolenza & DeRigne, 2019; Bolin & Kurtz, 2018). Significant distress can emerge for these communities as they fight to maintain their well-being and safety in the face of disaster-related loss, thus increasing their risk for negative mental health outcomes (Ford, 2009; Hobfoll & Ford, 2007).

Income is consistently linked to mental health outcomes following disasters (e.g., Ahern & Galea, 2006; Rhodes et al., 2010). For low-income communities, the cumulative impact of a disaster, coupled with place-based and environmental stressors rooted in historic and systemic inequality, can contribute to feelings of helplessness and loss of control, placing individuals at increased risk for mental health difficulties (Sandifer & Walker, 2018). When disasters strike, low-income communities have less access to disaster preparation, fewer recovery resources, and experience higher levels of displacement and forced residential changes (Elliott & Pais, 2006). These inequities directly contribute to worse post-disaster psychological recovery for low-income individuals (see Goldmann & Galea, 2014 for review). When Hurricane Katrina made landfall in 2005, Black residents tended to live in areas that sustained greater flooding damage than White residents. This resulted in more prolonged displacement and increased levels of psychological distress (Fussell et al., 2010; Fussell & Lowe, 2014).

Individuals belonging to marginalized ethnic and racial groups are also at heightened risk for mental health problems following disasters. This risk is likely linked to inequities rooted in historical and current xenophobia, racism, and classism. Ethnically and racially marginalized individuals are more likely to live in low-income communities due to geographic segregation and environmental racism (Bullard, 2000; Fussell et al., 2010), ingrained factors that exacerbated infection spread during the COVID-19 pandemic (Yang et al., 2021). Ethnically and racially marginalized communities also tend to be in closer proximity to environmental hazards and have less protective infrastructure compared to wealthier and Whiter communities (Reid, 2013). When exposed to disasters, ethnically and racially marginalized communities have access to fewer recovery resources, placing them at greater risk for mental health distress.

Age also impacts post-disaster mental health risk. Children are at increased risk due to their still-developing coping resources and reliance on adults (Lai & La Greca, 2020). Conversely, older adults (65+) may be at increased risk due to low rates of mental health service utilization, which may be linked to factors, including stigma and physical mobility (e.g., Wang et al., 2007), and a tendency to perceive disaster losses as particularly severe (Ashida et al., 2015; Friedsam, 1961; Tuohy et al., 2014). However, some research has found that older age is a protective factor against post-disaster mental health symptoms, which may be linked to previous experiences coping with disasters and/or trauma (Ngo, 2001).

To understand the impact of disasters on mental health, one must consider that people function within social systems (Cutter et al., 2003). Mental health risk is therefore created within systems that often fail to support the needs of vulnerable populations (Smiley et al., 2022). Disaster vulnerability is directly linked to systems that perpetuate inequity. Therefore, interventions aimed at alleviating the impact of disasters on mental health distress must address cumulative and intersectional risk factors that perpetuate vulnerability.

## PROTECTIVE FACTORS

Although the *absence* of the risk factors described above often implies protection (Akbar & Aldrich, 2018), this section will focus on additional factors that can protect individuals from psychopathology and promote positive adaptation. Biological, psychological, and social resources exert effects, often interacting, to improve post-disaster mental health (Hobfoll, 2001; Masten, 2019).

Regarding biological resources, neural circuit functioning and interactions between genes and the environment help mediate positive adaptation in human biopsychosocial systems after major stressors, such as disasters (Amstadter et al., 2014; Stein et al., 2019). For example, Gan et al. (2019) found that earthquake survivors carrying a particular genetic variation in the Neuropeptide Y gene showed resilience levels that were uniquely unaffected by higher trauma exposure.

Psychological resources also can promote positive post-disaster adaptation. Beginning with trait characteristics, greater resilience has been found to be associated with fewer symptoms of PTS and depressive symptoms (Bistricky et al., 2019). Self-compassion may also be protective, helping individuals manage difficult emotions, feel greater community solidarity, and boost perceived coping self-efficacy after a disaster (Lea et al., 2020). Coping self-efficacy, or an individual's belief in their ability to handle stressors, is associated with lower levels of distress and more effective coping behaviors (Benight et al., 1999; Bosmans et al., 2013). Active coping can reduce stressors and decrease the use of maladaptive coping strategies, such as avoidance, effectively reducing the likelihood of negative mental health outcomes (Pfefferbaum et al., 2014). Religious or spiritual coping can help individuals adapt to the impacts of disasters through creating meaning, receiving support from faith-based communities, and cultivating hope (de Castella & Simmonds, 2013; Shannonhouse et al., 2019), which may promote post-traumatic growth and well-being (Long et al., 2020).

Community support may appear in different forms, from faith-based communities to neighborhood hubs. Schools represent a community support that nurtures positive adaptation post-disaster. Schools can support families by providing emergency shelters, first-aid clinics, information, bonding, and security (Lai et al., 2016; Mutch, 2015). These types of support, as well as unity and membership within a community, provide a sense of collective identity, leading to positive outcomes for the entire community (Kaniasty et al., 2020; Littleton et al., 2022). Further, reinforcement of structures, food access, evacuation plans, and emergency personnel foster community preparedness for disasters, lessening the impacts of future disasters, particularly relevant for recurrently affected communities. In sum, fortifying and activating individual, family, and community resources can optimize populations' mental health and functioning before, during, and after a disaster.

## CASE EXAMPLE

"God willing, it will steer around us," says Sofia's elderly neighbor from behind his cloth mask as she hands him the pan. "We get it worst, but this is home," she says, and they nod. Both are part of a tight-knit, impoverished, and ethnically marginalized community in a highly populated coastal region, which regularly experiences hurricanes and floods. Sofia cares for her ailing mother, a 6-year-old daughter, and a 10-year-old son, who cannot forget the last major hurricane because of the still-boarded-up storefronts. The area where they live is largely ignored by the city, aside from what feels like round-the-clock police patrols. Their community bears accumulated wounds of neglect, mistreatment, and trauma. The current respiratory pandemic is straining psychological endurance, making it easy to ignore reports that a storm might arrive in a week. Sofia is more concerned about how to get her son to do his school homework while she works two jobs and runs the household.

Two days later, the storm gathered strength—a tropical storm, then a hurricane. It flattens islands on a trajectory toward Sofia's city. At home, Sofia and her mother track news coverage of destruction that has happened, is happening, and may happen. Stress is not good for Mom's hypertension and diabetes. Unfortunately, the storm regathers strength in warmer-than-usual waters, now certain to strike in the next 2 days. An evacuation order is issued, and rain begins to fall. By the time Sofia's supervisor allows her to leave and supplement her emergency preparation kit with toilet paper, water, and other essentials to ride out the storm, store shelves are bare. Mom's prescriptions only get half-filled. People are responding in a variety of ways: anxiety, confusion, acquiescence, and even bravado. Rain and wind intensity increase over the next 2 days.

Finally, it hits—torrential rain and 160 mile-per-hour winds. Power goes out, debris slams against Sofia's small home. Parts of the roof are torn off. Water is coming into the attic. No one in the family sleeps much that night. By early morning, the wind speed decreases, but water levels rise to the front door's threshold. Irreplaceable items are gathered and stuffed into a backpack. In short spells, Sofia feels outside her body and disoriented to time. Cellular networks are down, so Sofia can't call anyone. There is the smell and steady hum of gasoline generators, with occasional piercing sirens from afar. Two men with small rowboats ferry older adults from their homes. A Red Cross helicopter hovers nearby.

Within days, Sofia and her family are in a large makeshift shelter with hordes of others. They will not be able to access their house for weeks, and there is incessant coughing in the shelter. Is it from the pandemic or environmental toxins from the flooding? Sofia has an irritating rash all over her body, and she has been having nightmares. She must have witnessed her elderly neighbor being carried away by the flood water current, but she can only remember an intruding image and feels stuck in a moment of terror. She feels chronically keyed up, short-tempered, and overwhelmed. Why does *she* get to survive?

After a week, Sofia's extended family, who live further inland, politely refused a safe place to stay because they cannot risk it with their baby. She has also learned that both of her workplaces have suspended business indefinitely. After a few weeks living in the shelter, her extended family finally lets them move into a small, quarantined room. When Sofia and her children can finally survey their flooded home, the drywall is molded, and the air is unbreathable. Their home will need rebuilding—but how? Sofia has no income, work, childcare, or transportation, and disaster aid is hard to come by.

Time passes, news media move on, and the initial outpouring of resources dries up. Outside Sofia's community, one could get a (false) sense that life has returned to normal. Sofia tries to appear calm for her children, but she has begun to drink, as the anxiety, sadness, and desperation come in powerful waves. Sofia and her children remain disconnected from their spiritual community, enjoyable activities, and social relationships, making them wonder if life's biggest challenges are manageable.

More time passes, and Sofia and her children begin attending a place of worship in their new community that has few members from their culture. In struggling with distress and adversity, Sofia's damaged faith is taking a new and different form. Her son's early problems in his new school improve as he befriends another boy displaced by the hurricane. Sofia is also experiencing new forms of connection with those who welcomed her family. However, her mother's health has worsened. Sofia continues with uncertainty, with love and protection for her family, and with painful truths learned.

BRIEF ANALYSIS

In this example, we see intersecting risk and protective factors within the context of a *compound hazard*, demonstrating the mitigation conflict between maximizing shelter and minimizing exposure to infection from population crowding and mobility. Within the first 18 months of the COVID-19 pandemic, this conflict played out as 70 countries experienced floods. We also see the impacts of social support deterioration and emerging post-traumatic growth.

## THE FUTURE

Projections on disaster intensity, frequency, effects, and compound hazards will require understanding and shaping impacts through effective planning for each part of the disaster cycle: prevention and mitigation, preparedness, response, recovery, and rehabilitation (Simonovic et al., 2021). Methodologies in disaster research and disaster management must be interdisciplinary and integrate evolving technologies to maximize data quality in inherently difficult circumstances. For example, crowdsourcing and ecological momentary assessment can collect time-and-geolocated data through smartphones, multilevel modeling can be used to understand disaster-relevant behavior nested within communities, and advances in computer simulation and geographical information systems can help model complex processes and optimize strategic decision-making and communication across all phases of the disaster process (Donner & Diaz, 2018; Feinberg & Johnson, 1995; Laituri & Kodrich, 2008). The ability to mitigate surges of disaster-related mental health needs must be significantly increased (Everly, 2021). This would likely require leveraging existing community networks and peer support specialists alongside robust health systems to increase stress resistance, foster social support, encourage adaptive coping and cognition, and address other risk factors and protective factors reviewed in this chapter (Kaminsky et al., 2007). The goals would be to reduce symptoms and functional deterioration and to increase adaptation and potential for post-traumatic growth.

## CONCLUSION

Disasters are different from other forms of trauma, and thus they have different impacts. Disasters are collectively experienced, though the distribution of impact and resources to prepare for and mitigate impacts are typically unequal. Biopsychosocial risk and protective factors for various impacts exist at systemically interrelated individual, family, community, cultural, and societal levels. Interdisciplinary research and intervention will need to address these given that the impacts of disasters loom increasingly larger over humans' resilience and well-being, now and into the future.

# REFERENCES


Ahern, J., & Galea, S. (2006). Social context and depression after a disaster: The role of income inequality. *Journal of Epidemiology & Community Health*, 60(9), 766–770. https://doi.org/10.1136/jech.2006.042069

Akbar, M. S., & Aldrich, D. P. (2018). Social capital's role in recovery: Evidence from communities affected by the 2010 Pakistan floods. *Disasters*, 42(3), 475–497. https://doi.org/10.1111/disa.12259

Alcántara, C., & Lewis- Fernández, R. (2016). Chapter 8. Latinas' and Latinos' risk for PTSD after trauma exposure: A review of sociocultural explanations. In D. E. Hinton & B. J. Good (Eds.), *Culture and PTSD* (pp. 275–306). University of Pennsylvania Press. https://doi.org/10.9783/9780812291469-009

Amstadter, A. B., Myers, J. M., & Kendler, K. S. (2014). Psychiatric resilience: Longitudinal twin study. *British Journal of Psychiatry*, 205(4), 275–280. https://doi.org/10.1192/bjp.bp.113.130906

APA (2022). *DSM-5-TR classification*. American Psychiatric Association Publishing.

Ashida, S., Robinson, E. L., Gay, J., & Ramirez, M. (2015). Motivating rural older residents to prepare for disasters: Moving beyond personal benefits. *Ageing and Society*, 36(10), 2117–2140. https://doi.org/10.1017/S0144686X15000914

Baggerly, J., Ceballos, P., Rodríguez, M., & Reyes, A. G. (2022). Cultural adaptations for disaster response for children in Puerto Rico after Hurricane María. *Journal of Multicultural Counseling and Development*, 50(3), 118–127. https://doi.org/10.1002/jmcd.12246

Benevolenza, M. A., & DeRigne, L. (2019). The impact of climate change and natural disasters on vulnerable populations: A systematic review of literature. *Journal of Human Behavior in the Social Environment*, 29(2), 266–281. https://doi.org/10.1080/10911359.2018.1527739

Benight, C. C., Swift, E., Sanger, J., Smith, A., & Zeppelin, D. (1999). Coping self-efficacy as a mediator of distress following a natural disaster. *Journal of Applied Social Psychology*, 29(12), 2443–2464. https://doi.org/10.1111/j.1559-1816.1999.tb00120.x

Bistricky, S. L., Long, L. J., Lai, B. S., Gallagher, M. W., Kanenberg, H., Elkins, S. R., Harper, K. L., & Short, M. B. (2019). Surviving the storm: Avoidant coping, helping behavior, resilience and affective symptoms around a major hurricane-flood. *Journal of Affective Disorders*, 257, 297–306. https://doi.org/10.1016/j.jad.2019.07.044

Bolin, R., & Kurtz, L. C. (2018). Race, class, ethnicity, and disaster vulnerability. In H. Rodríguez, W. Donner, & J. E. Trainor (Eds.), *Handbook of disaster research* (pp. 181–203). Springer International Publishing. https://doi.org/10.1007/978-3-319-63254-4_10

Bosmans, M. W. G., Benight, C. C., van der Knaap, L. M., Winkel, F. W., & van der Velden, P. G. (2013). The associations between coping self-efficacy and posttraumatic stress symptoms 10 years post-disaster: Differences between men and women. *Journal of Traumatic Stress, 26*(1), 184–191. https://doi.org/10.1002/jts.21789

Bullard, R. D. (2000). *Dumping in Dixie: Race, class, and environmental quality* (3rd ed.). Westview Press.

de Castella, R., & Simmonds, J. G. (2013). "There's a deeper level of meaning as to what suffering's all about": Experiences of religious and spiritual growth following trauma. *Mental Health, Religion and Culture, 16*(5), 536–556. https://doi.org/10.1080/13674676.2012.702738

Cutter, S. L., Boruff, B. J., & Shirley, W. L. (2003). Social vulnerability to environmental hazards. *Social Science Quarterly, 84*(2), 242–261. https://doi.org/10.1111/1540-6237.8402002

Donner, W., & Diaz, W. (2018). Methodological issues in disaster research. In H. Rodríguez, W. Donner, & J. E. Trainor (Eds.), *Handbook of disaster research* (pp. 289–309). Springer International Publishing. https://doi.org/10.1007/978-3-319-63254-4_15

Elliott, J. R., & Pais, J. (2006). Race, class, and Hurricane Katrina: Social differences in responses to disaster. *Social Science Research, 35*(2), 295–321. https://doi.org/10.1016/j.ssresearch.2006.02.003

Everly, G. S. (2021). Disaster mental health: Remembering the past, shaping the future. *International Review of Psychiatry, 33*(8), 663–667. https://doi.org/10.1080/09540261.2022.2031633

Feinberg, W. E., & Johnson, N. R. (1995). FIRESCAP: A computer simulation model of reaction to a fire alarm. *The Journal of Mathematical Sociology, 20*(2–3), 247–269. https://doi.org/10.1080/0022250X.1995.9990164

Ford, J. D. (2009). Prevention of traumatic stress disorders. In *Posttraumatic stress disorder* (pp. 251–279). Elsevier. https://doi.org/10.1016/B978-0-12-374462-3.00009-5

Friedsam, H. J. (1961). Reactions of older persons to disaster-caused losses: An hypothesis of relative deprivation. *The Gerontologist, 1*(1), 34–37. https://doi.org/10.1093/geront/1.1.34

Furr, J. M., Comer, J. S., Edmunds, J. M., & Kendall, P. C. (2010). Disasters and youth: A meta-analytic examination of posttraumatic stress. *Journal of Consulting and Clinical Psychology, 78*(6), 765–780. https://doi.org/10.1037/a0021482

Fussell, E., & Lowe, S. R. (2014). The impact of housing displacement on the mental health of low-income parents after Hurricane Katrina. *Social Science & Medicine, 113*(1), 137–144. https://doi.org/10.1016/j.socscimed.2014.05.025

Fussell, E., Sastry, N., & VanLandingham, M. (2010). Race, socioeconomic status, and return migration to New Orleans after Hurricane Katrina. *Population and Environment, 31*(1–3), 20–42. https://doi.org/10.1007/s11111-009-0092-2

Galatzer-Levy, I. R., Huang, S. H., & Bonanno, G. A. (2018). Trajectories of resilience and dysfunction following potential trauma: A review and statistical evaluation. *Clinical Psychology Review, 63*, 41–55. https://doi.org/10.1016/j.cpr.2018.05.008

Gan, Y., Chen, Y., Han, X., Yu, N. X., & Wang, L. (2019). Neuropeptide Y gene × environment interaction predicts resilience and positive future focus. *Applied Psychology. Health and Well-Being, 11*(3), 438–458. https://doi.org/10.1111/aphw.12162

García, F. E., Cova, F., Rincón, P., & Vázquez, C. (2015). Trauma or growth after a natural disaster? The mediating role of rumination processes. *European Journal of Psychotraumatology, 6*(1), 26557. https://doi.org/10.3402/ejpt.v6.26557

Goldmann, E., & Galea, S. (2014). Mental health consequences of disasters. *Annual Review of Public Health, 35*(1), 169–183. https://doi.org/10.1146/annurev-publhealth-032013-182435

Hobfoll, S. E. (2001). The influence of culture, community, and the nested-self in the stress process: Advancing conservation of resources theory. *Applied Psychology, 50*(3), 337–421. https://doi.org/10.1111/1464-0597.00062

Hobfoll, S. E., & Ford, J. S. (2007). Conservation of resources theory. In G. Fink (Ed.), *Encyclopedia of stress* (pp. 562–567). Elsevier. https://doi.org/10.1016/B978-012373947-6.00093-3

Kaminsky, M., McCabe, O. L., Langlieb, A. M., & Everly, G. S. (2007). An evidence-informed model of human resistance, resilience, and recovery: The Johns Hopkins' outcome-driven paradigm for disaster mental health services. *Brief Treatment and Crisis Intervention, 7*(1), 1–11. https://doi.org/10.1093/brief-treatment/mhl015

Kaniasty, K., de Terte, I., Guilaran, J., & Bennett, S. (2020). A scoping review of post-disaster social support investigations conducted after disasters that struck the Australia and Oceania continent. *Disasters, 44*(2), 336–366. https://doi.org/10.1111/disa.12390

Lai, B. S., & La Greca, A. (2020). *Understanding the impacts of natural disasters on children* [Child Evidence Brief].

Lai, B. S., La Greca, A. M., Auslander, B. A., & Short, M. B. (2013). Children's symptoms of posttraumatic stress and depression after a natural disaster: Comorbidity and risk factors. *Journal of Affective Disorders, 146*(1), 71–78. https://doi.org/10.1016/j.jad.2012.08.041

Lai, B. S., Esnard, A.-M., Lowe, S. R., & Peek, L. (2016). Schools and disasters: Safety and mental health assessment and interventions for children. *Current Psychiatry Reports, 18*(12), 109. https://doi.org/10.1007/s11920-016-0743-9

Lai, B. S., La Greca, A. M., Brincks, A., Colgan, C. A., D'Amico, M. P., Lowe, S., & Kelley, M. L. (2021). Trajectories of posttraumatic stress in youths after natural disasters. *JAMA Network Open, 4*(2), e2036682. https://doi.org/10.1001/jamanetworkopen.2020.36682

Laituri, M., & Kodrich, K. (2008). On Line disaster response community: People as sensors of high magnitude disasters using internet GIS. *Sensors, 8*(5), 3037–3055. https://doi.org/10.3390/s8053037

Lea, C. S., Littleton, H., Allen, A. B., & Beasley, C. M. (2020). Resilience, self-compassion, and mental health outcomes: Rebuilding eastern North Carolina after natural disasters. *North Carolina Medical Journal, 81*(5), 315–319. https://doi.org/10.18043/ncm.81.5.315

Lee, J.-Y., Kim, S.-W., & Kim, J.-M. (2020). The impact of community disaster trauma: A focus on emerging research of PTSD and other mental health outcomes. *Chonnam Medical Journal, 56*(2), 99. https://doi.org/10.4068/cmj.2020.56.2.99

Littleton, H., Haney, L., Schoemann, A., Allen, A., & Benight, C. (2022). Received support in the aftermath of Hurricane Florence: Reciprocal relations among perceived support, community solidarity, and PTSD. *Anxiety, Stress, and Coping, 35*(3), 270–283. https://doi.org/10.1080/10615806.2021.1956480

Long, L. J., Bistricky, S. L., Phillips, C. A., D'Souza, J. M., Richardson, A. L., Lai, B. S., Short, M., & Gallagher, M. W. (2020). The potential unique impacts of hope and resilience on mental health and well-being in the wake of Hurricane Harvey. *Journal of Traumatic Stress, 33*(6), 962–972. https://doi.org/10.1002/jts.22555

Lowe, S. R., McGrath, J. A., Young, M. N., Kwok, R. K., Engel, L. S., Galea, S., & Sandler, D. P. (2019). Cumulative disaster exposure and mental and physical health symptoms among a large sample of Gulf Coast residents. *Journal of Traumatic Stress, 32*(2), 196–205. https://doi.org/10.1002/jts.22392

Lowe, S. R., Ratanatharathorn, A., Lai, B. S., van der Mei, W., Barbano, A. C., Bryant, R. A., Delahanty, D. L., Matsuoka, Y. J., Olff, M., Schnyder, U., Laska, E., Koenen, K. C., Shalev, A. Y., & Kessler, R. C. (2021). Posttraumatic stress disorder symptom trajectories within the first year following emergency department admissions: Pooled results from the International Consortium to predict PTSD. *Psychological Medicine, 51*(7), 1129–1139. https://doi.org/10.1017/S0033291719004008

Masten, A. S. (2019). Resilience from a developmental systems perspective. *World Psychiatry, 18*(1), 101–102. https://doi.org/10.1002/wps.20591

Mayena, B. S., O'Brien, G., O'Keefe, P., & Rose, J. (2011). Disaster resilience: A bounce back or bounce forward ability? *Local Environment, 16*(5), 417–424. https://doi.org/10.1080/13549839.2011.583049

Mutch, C. (2015). The role of schools in disaster settings: Learning from the 2010–2011 New Zealand earthquakes. *International Journal of Educational Development, 41,* 283–291. https://doi.org/10.1016/j.ijedudev.2014.06.008

Neria, Y., Nandi, A., & Galea, S. (2008). Post-traumatic stress disorder following disasters: A systematic review. *Psychological Medicine, 38*(4), 467–480. https://doi.org/10.1017/S0033291707001353

Newnham, E. A., Mergelsberg, E. L. P., Chen, Y., Kim, Y., Gibbs, L., Dzidic, P. L., Ishida DaSilva, M., Chan, E. Y. Y., Shimomura, K., Narita, Z., Huang, Z., & Leaning, J. (2022). Long term mental health trajectories after disasters and pandemics: A multilingual systematic review of prevalence, risk and protective factors. *Clinical Psychology Review, 97,* 102203. https://doi.org/10.1016/j.cpr.2022.102203

Ngo, E. B. (2001). When disasters and age collide: Reviewing vulnerability of the elderly. *Natural Hazards Review, 2*(2), 80–89. https://doi.org/10.1061/(ASCE)1527-6988(2001)2:2(80)

Ornes, S. (2018). How does climate change influence extreme weather? Impact attribution research seeks answers. *Proceedings of the National Academy of Sciences, 115*(33), 8232–8235. https://doi.org/10.1073/pnas.1811393115

Pfefferbaum, B., Noffsinger, M. A., Wind, L. H., & Allen, J. R. (2014). Children's coping in the context of disasters and terrorism. *Journal of Loss and Trauma, 19*(1), 78–97. https://doi.org/10.1080/15325024.2013.791797

Qassem, T., Aly-El Gabry, D., Alzarouni, A., Abdel-Aziz, K., & Arnone, D. (2021). Psychiatric co-morbidities in post-traumatic stress disorder: Detailed findings from the Adult Psychiatric Morbidity Survey in the English population. *Psychiatric Quarterly, 92*(1), 321–330. https://doi.org/10.1007/s11126-020-09797-4

Rahmani, M., Muzwagi, A., & Pumariega, A. J. (2022). Cultural factors in disaster response among diverse children and youth around the world. *Current Psychiatry Reports, 24*(10), 481–491. https://doi.org/10.1007/s11920-022-01356-x

Reid, M. (2013). Disasters and social inequalities: Disasters and social inequalities. *Sociology Compass, 7*(11), 984–997. https://doi.org/10.1111/soc4.12080

Rhodes, J., Chan, C., Paxson, C., Rouse, C. E., Waters, M., & Fussell, E. (2010). The impact of Hurricane Katrina on the mental and physical health of low-income parents in New Orleans. *American Journal of Orthopsychiatry, 80*(2), 237–247. https://doi.org/10.1111/j.1939-0025.2010.01027.x

Sandifer, P. A., & Walker, A. H. (2018). Enhancing disaster resilience by reducing stress-associated health impacts. *Frontiers in Public Health, 6*(373), 1–20. https://www.frontiersin.org/articles/10.3389/fpubh.2018.00373/full

Self-Brown, S., Lai, B., Patterson, A., & Glasheen, T. (2017). The impact of natural disasters on youth: A focus on emerging research beyond internalizing disorders. *Current Psychiatry Reports, 19*(53), 1–7. https://doi.org/10.1007/s11920-017-0798-2

Shannonhouse, L. R., Bialo, J. A., Majuta, A. R., Zeligman, M. R., Davis, D. E., McElroy-Heltzel, S. E., Aten, J. D., Davis, E. B., Van Tongeren, D. R., & Hook, J. N. (2019). Conserving resources during chronic disaster: Impacts of religious and meaning-focused coping on Botswana drought survivors. *Psychological Trauma Theory Research Practice and Policy, 11*(2), 137–146. https://doi.org/10.1037/tra0000420

Simonovic, S. P., Kundzewicz, Z. W., & Wright, N. (2021). Floods and the COVID -19 pandemic—A new double hazard problem. *WIREs Water, 8*(2). https://doi.org/10.1002/wat2.1509

Smiley, K. T., Domingue, S. J., Lewis, A. L., McNeese, H., Pellegrin, S. J., & Sandhu, H. (2022). Inequalities and interrelations: The sociology of disasters at a new crossroads. *Sociology Compass, 16*(12). https://doi.org/10.1111/soc4.13008

Smith, A. B. (2020, January 8). 2010–2019: A landmark decade of U.S. billion-dollar weather and climate disasters. In *Beyond the Data*. https://www.climate.gov/news-features/blogs/beyond-data/2010-2019-landmark-decade-us-billion-dollar-weather-and-climate

Stein, M. B., Choi, K. W., Jain, S., Campbell-Sills, L., Chen, C., Gelernter, J., He, F., Heeringa, S. G., Maihofer, A. X., Nievergelt, C., Nock, M. K., Ripke, S., Sun, X., Kessler, R. C., Smoller, J. W., & Ursano, R. J. (2019). Genome-wide analyses of psychological resilience in U.S. Army soldiers. *American Journal of Medical Genetics Part B: Neuropsychiatric Genetics, 180*(5), 310–319. https://doi.org/10.1002/ajmg.b.32730

Tedeschi, R. G., Shakespeare-Finch, J., Taku, K., & Calhoun, L. G. (2018). *Posttraumatic growth: Theory, research, and applications* (1st ed.). Routledge. https://doi.org/10.4324/9781315527451

Thiery, W., Lange, S., Rogelj, J., Schleussner, C.-F., Gudmundsson, L., Seneviratne, S. I., Andrijevic, M., Frieler, K., Emanuel, K., Geiger, T., Bresch, D. N., Zhao, F., Willner, S. N., Büchner, M., Volkholz, J., Bauer, N., Chang, J., Ciais, P., Dury, M., . . . Wada, Y. (2021). Intergenerational inequities in exposure to climate extremes. *Science, 374*(6564), 158–160. https://doi.org/10.1126/science.abi7339

Tuohy, R., Stephens, C., & Johnston, D. (2014). Older adults' disaster preparedness in the context of the September 2010–December 2012 Canterbury earthquake sequence. *International Journal of Disaster Risk Reduction, 9*(1), 194–203. https://doi.org/10.1016/j.ijdrr.2014.05.010

Wang, P. S., Gruber, M. J., Powers, R. E., Schoenbaum, M., Speier, A. H., Wells, K. B., & Kessler, R. C. (2007). Mental health service use among Hurricane Katrina survivors in the eight months after the disaster. *Psychiatric Services*, *58*(11), 1403–1411. https://doi.org/10.1176/ps.2007.58.11.1403

Yang, T., Choi, S. E., & Sun, F. (2021). COVID-19 cases in US counties: Roles of racial/ethnic density and residential segregation. *Ethnicity & Health*, *26*(1), 11–21. https://doi.org/10.1080/13557858.2020.1830036

## CHAPTER NINE

# Trauma-Informed Considerations with Neurodivergent Children and Adolescents

ROBERT JASON GRANT and RACHEL WETHERS

## NEURODIVERGENT CHILDREN AND ADOLESCENTS

Neurodiversity is the idea that neurological differences such as autism, attention-deficit hyperactivity disorder (ADHD), learning differences, and sensory differences, are the result of normal, natural variation in the human genome (Robinson, 2018). Grant (2023) stated that underneath the "umbrella" of neurodiversity, there currently exist two primary categories of people—neurodivergent and neurotypical—to understand the definition of one is to understand the definition of the other. Neurotypical describes individuals who display a society-defined typical intellectual and social development. Neurodivergent refers to individuals who have a less typical (society considered "not normal") intellectual and social variation, such as but not limited to autism, ADHD, dyslexia, dyspraxia, dyscalculia, sensory differences, obsessive-compulsive disorder (OCD), intellectual developmental disorder, Tourette's Syndrome, and so on.

Being neurodivergent is often first recognized as the result of a diagnosis, but neurodivergence can exist before and without a diagnosis. It is possible to become neurodivergent as the result of physical or emotional injury or trauma, but in most cases, neurodivergence typically exists from birth

*Trauma Impacts: The Repercussions of Individual and Collective Trauma*, First Edition.
Edited by Jessica Stone, Robert J. Grant, and Clair Mellenthin.
© 2024 John Wiley & Sons, Inc. Published 2024 by John Wiley & Sons, Inc.

onward. For each neurodivergent child, there exists a spectrum of presentation, which makes each child unique. Neurodivergent individuals do share commonalities and some differences from the neuronormative in processing, communication, social navigation, sensory processing, emotion recognition, expression, learning, and so on (Grant, 2023). For the purpose of this chapter, we will present trauma-related information, conceptualizing the general experiences of neurodivergent children and adolescents.

## NEURODIVERGENCE AND TRAUMA

Neurodivergent children can experience a traumatic event or be affected by trauma, including meeting the criteria for a trauma disorder (Ryder, 2022). Research supports that neurodivergent children experience traumatic events and can experience trauma reactions and trauma-related disorders at the same percentage (and often higher) as neurotypical children (Hoover, 2015). Research further indicates that autistic children show an increase in anxiety-related chemicals (particularly cortisol), in response to stressors, triggering more quickly and intensely than in neurotypical individuals (Spratt et al., 2012). Due to this increase, an autistic child may have a stronger reaction to a trauma event than a neurotypical child would have.

It is important to understand neurodivergence as a trauma response. The everyday life experiences of neurodivergent children tend to make them vulnerable to experiencing trauma simply because they are neurodivergent and navigating in a predominately ableist society. Neurodivergent children experience their environments in heightened ways. Their social experiences are perceived through a lens unique to them. Due to nervous systems that can become dysregulated by a variety of experiences, they are more likely to notice traumas and experience them more deeply on a biological level. Regulating stress reactions can be more difficult for those who are neurodivergent. Research has identified that neurodivergent neurobiology is more vulnerable and reactive with a differing parasympathetic response system (Beauchaine et al., 2013).

Neurodivergence as a trauma response means trying to navigate a world that is inherently rejecting the way you think, process, learn, and experience. Neurodivergent individuals are often forced to participate in a neurotypical climate that has been deemed the correct and expected way, with little acceptance of differences. Being told that you are less than, lacking, odd, something is wrong with you, not good enough, and/or need to be "worked on," "fixed," or "cured" can—and often does—create trauma for the neurodivergent child (Gates, 2019; Robinson, 2018).

Many neurodivergent children have sensory processing challenges. When a person is constantly under sensory assault, their regulatory system becomes overwhelmed, and eventually creates a trauma response. Additionally, many of the symptoms of the under-responsive sensory individual have been noted in trauma survivors. This can be attributed to cases of extreme trauma where survivors disconnect themselves from body awareness that could trigger trauma memory and sensation, which makes them under responsive to sensory integration (Cox, 2016; Grant, 2022; Hurim et al., 2016).

Research exploring peer victimization and bullying often highlights the potential traumatization of autistic children and adolescents, as autistic children are more often bullied than peers with other disabilities, as well as those who are non-disabled (Guest & Ohrt, 2018). Estimates from a variety of studies (Hoover, 2015) indicate that parent and children surveys report 44–77% of autistic children being bullied within a one-month period, as compared to a rate of 2–17% in surveys focused on neurotypically developing children. Another large parent survey (Hoover, 2015) suggested that as many as 94% of autistic children and children with other nonverbal learning disorders are bullied at some point within a 12-month period.

Autistic and other neurodivergent children are more susceptible to victimization and experience traumatic effects differently than other children, and they may perceive daily common events as traumatic due to their varied perceptions and sensitivity to stimuli (Guest & Ohrt, 2018). Children with intellectual and developmental disabilities are 1.5 to 3 times more likely than their peers to experience maltreatment resulting in trauma issues. These children are likely to be more dependent on adults and may have difficulty communicating their experiences of harm, thus continuing to be victimized without receiving support (Kerns et al., 2020).

Neurodivergent children and adolescents can develop post-traumatic stress disorder (PTSD) and other trauma disorders due to many factors. The common co-occurring difficulties related to various mental health or developmental needs can include language and communication barriers, which, at times, make it difficult for them to report traumatic experiences to their reliable adults (Fisher et al., 2022; Haruvi-Lamdan et al., 2020). Up to 45% of autistic individuals are reported to have experienced PTSD, which is substantially higher than the 4% prevalence rate approximated for the general population (Fisher et al., 2022). Up to 17% of trauma-exposed children meet ADHD criteria, and the co-occurrence increases problematic needs related to both trauma and ADHD (Brown, 2022).

Stigma is also a form of trauma. It targets people on the basis of beliefs about them that have nothing to do with who they are. It undermines a person's humanity and overshadows the fullness of their identity. When a person's humanity is threatened, undermined, and devalued, it is fundamentally traumatic. It can shift a person into a hyperarousal state of defensive safety-seeking or guarded withdrawal and self-isolation. This kind of trauma in neurodivergence can be experienced as shame, rejection, and/or devaluation, which is often the result of ableism (Gates, 2019).

Over time, neurodivergent individuals can accumulate many experiences of social rejection and isolation, resulting in a fear of social situations and an anxiety/trauma response when entering social situations (Robinson, 2018). Often autistic and other neurodivergent individuals are judged, dismissed, marginalized, rejected, stereotyped, spoken for, and have their "voice" taken away by neurotypical individuals. A neurodivergent individual's social value is often diminished because their actions do not conform to conventional standards. Environments are designed by and for neurotypical individuals with little to no thought given to those with differing abilities, preferences, or needs. Even "therapies" intended to help can create trauma. The history of treatments and therapies has not been very affirming and has often treated autistic and other neurodivergent children as problematic or as a disease to be cured. This type of thinking and approach has been detrimental to the neurodivergent individual's self-worth and value. Repeated exposure to non-affirming treatments can produce a trauma response. (Anderson, 2022)

## ADVERSE CHILDHOOD EXPERIENCES

Fuld (2018) determined that adverse childhood experiences (ACEs) directly lead to stress and trauma, and those who are neurodivergent have a "significantly higher probability" (than those who are not neurodivergent) of experiencing one or more ACEs in their childhood. ACEs are reported more frequently by families of autistic children, particularly experiences of parental divorce and income insufficiency (Kerns et al., 2017). Therapists working with neurodivergent children will need to consider what (if any) ACEs exist and may be contributing to presenting issues and trauma-related symptomology.

As observed in the general population, autistic children who experience an increased number of ACEs are at an elevated risk for comorbid psychiatric and medical health problems. Autistic children with an elevated number of ACEs often experience delays in diagnosis and treatment initiation (Hoover & Kaufman, 2018). Guest and Ohrt (2018) found that in a sample of 69 students diagnosed with autism, 26% had a history of trauma. Im (2016) reported that in a larger sample of 156 autistic students, 18.5% had a history of physical abuse, and 16.6% had been sexually abused, and the experience of this abuse was linked to trauma-related issues.

Unique characteristics of co-occurring adverse experiences also exist with ADHD reports. Children with ADHD are reported to have higher rates of each ACE type compared to children without ADHD (Brown et al., 2017). As ACE scores increase, the reported risk of also having ADHD rises, and the severity of ADHD also increases. Additionally, ACE-related issues such as socioeconomic hardship and having a caregiver with a mental illness, significantly increase the odds of a child having moderate-to-severe ADHD (Brown, 2022).

The potential to overlook neurodevelopmental conditions is particularly high if the child is experiencing adversity, and the existence of ACEs can delay the diagnosis of neurodivergent conditions. It is important to maintain a focus on both ACEs and neurodevelopmental conditions, since not doing so can place individuals in double jeopardy of poor health outcomes (Gajwani & Minnis, 2023).

## CONSIDERATIONS WITH NEURODIVERGENT CLIENTS

### INTERSECTIONALITY

Intersectionality recognizes how the complex and multifaceted nature of people's identities, including other disabilities, race, ethnicity, gender, sexuality, and class, impacts experiences and development across the lifespan. Diagnoses and support can rely upon these intersecting identities to produce unique, intersecting, interactional, and additive spaces of marginalization. Neurodivergent children and adolescents who are diverse in multiple ways, such as racial, ethnic, sexual, and/or gender minorities, may face unique and increased stigma and barriers to inclusion, that may lead to re-experiencing trauma symptoms. Neurodivergent people of color, women, trans, and/or nonbinary people, and people with fewer resources are often underdiagnosed with trauma and other needs, underserved, and underrepresented (Botha & Gillespie-Lynch, 2022).

The diversity awareness of neurodivergent individuals can be conceptualized within the greater diversity awareness paradigm. An understanding of racism, discrimination, prejudice, bigotry, and so on provides a greater understanding of what neurodiversity means. Walker (2021) proposed the importance of understanding neurodiversity as a natural form of human diversity, subject to the same societal dynamics as other forms of diversity. Diversity awareness also informs how neurodivergent people and their allies lead efforts in the neurodiversity movement to help improve acceptance and inclusion in societies that have historically lacked neurodivergent affirming constructs (Grant, 2023).

Studies show that individuals who experience microaggressions and persistent racism also demonstrate sustained toxic stress responses. Children of color are at increased risk of living in concentrated poverty, which is tied to moderate and severe ADHD diagnoses (Brown, 2022). A study of 170 Black, Latino, and multiracial gay and bisexual men found that the interaction between racial discrimination and gay rejection sensitivity explained higher levels of emotional regulation difficulties, which in turn predicted higher symptoms of anxiety, depression, and possible trauma symptoms (Botha & Gillespie-Lynch, 2022).

Neurodivergent sexual minorities are exposed to many forms of discrimination, including heteronormativity, homophobia, biphobia, and queerphobia, which are associated with worsened mental and physical health, including higher suicidality (Walker, 2021). Trans, nonbinary, and intersex people experience pervasive gender normativity, transphobia, and exorsexism (the assumption that gender and sex only exist in a male/female binary). Greater exposure to these minority stressors is related to worse well-being, higher psychological distress, and suicidality (Botha & Gillespie-Lynch, 2022).

The often-limited degree to which neurodivergent people with additional marginalized identities are represented by existing neurotypical advocacy efforts, research, and practice is a major concern. Those with marginalized identities often experience socio-cultural stigma and disadvantages, which both shape and are shaped by their identities. Collectively, we are only beginning to grapple with the degree to which intersectionality has been neglected in neurodiversity-affirming practice, research, and activism (Botha & Gillespie-Lynch, 2022).


## Disability and Ableism

Ableism is deeply ingrained in the fabric of most societies and systems, and continually fuels devaluing and traumatizing actions and stigmas that often go unchallenged. Eisenmenger (2019) described ableism as the discrimination and social prejudice against disabled people based on the belief that typical abilities are superior. Similar to racism and sexism, ableism classifies entire groups of people as "less than" and includes harmful stereotypes, misconceptions, and generalizations about disabled people. Ableism has been problematic and traumatic for many who have experienced it, as far back (and further even than) the Eugenics movement (a belief in creating perfect human beings and eliminating so-called social ills through genetics and heredity) in the early 1900s.

Ableism can encompass many things, including a lack of compliance with the Americans with Disabilities Act (ADA), segregating students with disabilities into alternative schools, the use of restraint or seclusion as a means of control, and/or failing to make websites and facilities accessible to all individuals. It also includes the assumption that a person might want to be "fixed" or would be happier without their disability. Being ableist can be as simple as not educating oneself on disability-inclusive language and ignoring the preferences of disability groups. Much like other stereotypes and adversities noted above, ableism is harmful and can produce long-lasting trauma effects such as debilitating anxiety, poor emotion modulation, social fears, and poor self-worth (Grant, 2023).

Many ableist actions tend to be in the form of microaggressions (slights, insults, putdowns, invalidations, and offensive behaviors that people experience in daily interactions). While not overt, these processes can still produce trauma in neurodivergent and disabled people. Internalized ableism is also a form of trauma. It leads to emotional difficulties, anger, resentment, relationship problems, and a refusal of neurodivergent individuals to accept themselves. Due to these issues, autistic and neurodivergent people are likely to develop a host of mental health needs such as depression, anxiety, substance abuse problems, and trauma (Lowry, n.d.).

## ALEXITHYMIA AND APHANTASIA

Affective modulation support is often necessary when working with neurodivergent children and adolescents addressing trauma needs. The goal of affective modulation support is to increase the capacity to identify a range of feelings, name the feelings, and identify appropriate expressions (Kirk et al., 2022). At times, pushing neurodivergent individuals to express and communicate their feelings in neurotypical ways can lead to emotional flooding, overwhelm, and shutdown for self-protection. Neurodivergent individuals utilize emotional awareness and expression in their own individual ways. Alexithymia, the difficulty of identifying or expressing emotions in neurotypical ways (Zackheim, 2007) and aphantasia, the difficulty of visualizing information (Dance et al., 2022), are common experiences of many neurodivergent people. Some clients may want to explore expanding these affective skills, and some may not. Self-determination is recognized in this area as vital in the therapeutic process with neurodivergent individuals. Often their voices are not heard or valued, and they should be an active part of therapeutic decisions and goals.

For neurodivergent individuals who prefer to not expand these skills, it is common that the person has discovered individualized ways to relate to their emotions. This has likely manifested through their struggles to view or understand emotions in neurotypical ways, which can leave them frustrated, demand avoidant, and/or shutting down. Alexithymia and aphantasia issues are important to understand as they may present specific awareness about the neurodivergent client and can inform how trauma issues are treated.

## NEURODIVERGENT TRAUMA-INFORMED INTERVENTIONS

When treating trauma in neurodivergent children, it is important to stay flexible and adapt to the child's needs and learning styles. Many neurodivergent individuals may present with a combination of adverse life events and psychiatric comorbidities. The therapist will need to adjust therapeutic goals to meet the uniqueness of each client and be willing to modify them throughout the course of treatment as applicable.

Neurologically, neurodivergent children often process information differently than neurotypical individuals. Processing speed, cognitive awareness, receptive language ability, and executive functioning ability may present differently (thorough and deliberate, concrete, visually, etc.) from a neurotypical person (Grant, 2023). This will affect how the therapy "looks," how it progresses, and what techniques or modalities the therapist might implement with the child. These factors must be taken into consideration when attempting to address trauma issues, especially when using trauma models developed for the neurotypical population such as Trauma Focused-Cognitive Behavioral Therapy (TF-CBT) and Eye Movement Desensitization and Reprocessing (EMDR). Most trauma protocols, trauma models, trauma treatments, and trauma assessment measures have been normed, validated, and researched with neurotypical individuals, not considering the neurodivergent presentation (Gates, 2019).

Despite an increasing evidence base regarding psychological therapies for neurodivergent children and adolescents, gaps remain between research and clinical practice. Neurodivergent individuals and their families consistently describe systemic barriers to accessing mental health support, including psychological therapy, service provisions (e.g., triage systems poorly aligned to social communication differences and capping of sessions irrespective of need), practitioners (e.g., limited knowledge about neurodivergence and uncertainty about how to adapt therapy), and characteristics of neurodivergence that may make accessing therapy more challenging (e.g., executive function difficulties, social communication differences, and sensory overwhelm) (Fisher et al., 2022).

Various trauma-informed therapies are used as modalities and tools to appropriately meet the needs of children and adolescents. The California Evidence-Based Clearinghouse for Child Welfare (2022), or CEBC, rates various theoretical approaches as appropriate trauma-informed interventions for children who experience high ACE backgrounds. The top three clinical modalities respected and preferred by the CEBC in 2022 and rated as level 1 or "well supported by research evidence," are EMDR, Prolonged Exposure Therapy for adolescents, and TF-CBT. Other theoretical modalities and interventions are rated within their system for additional review.

In general, two categories of approaches exist when addressing trauma—top–down approaches and bottom–up approaches. The brain is understood to generally develop "bottom–up," so when trauma occurs at much younger ages, we know bottom–up development is affected, and often bottom–up theoretical approaches are more effective with these youth.

Bottom–up therapies access earlier developed portions of the autonomic nervous system and emotion and memory storage and processing through the brain stem and limbic system. They often address instinctive responses and somatic awareness that is known to have begun development as early as prenatal stages. Common bottom–up approaches include Brainspotting, EMDR, Somatic Experiencing, Yoga, and other approaches such as Art Therapy, Play Therapy, AutPlay Therapy, and Sandtray Therapy (Reagan, 2021). It is also noted that mindfulness-based therapies are often discussed as having aspects of both top–down and bottom–up approaches. For adolescents who are older when trauma is experienced, "top–down" approaches may be preferred (Lyons, 2019). Top–down therapies are approaches rooted in recognizing, processing, and integrating cognitive frameworks. They rely on prefrontal cortex development and processing, which involves thinking and logic, cognitive emotional awareness, problem solving, and language, which often develop in the early stages of development at younger ages. These theoretical approaches often include but are not limited to popular approaches such as Cognitive Behavioral Therapy (CBT), Cognitive Processing Therapy, TF-CBT, Dialectical Behavioral Therapy (DBT), Acceptance and Commitment Therapy (ACT), Prolonged Exposure Therapy, Psychodynamic Therapy, Narrative Therapy, and Internal Family Systems Therapy (Reagan, 2021).

Neurodivergent children and adolescents of all ages may gravitate toward one or the other approaches, given their preferences in learning and exploration styles. It is vital to remember that no one therapy proven to be "the best therapy" for all neurodivergent individuals. Some neurodivergent children and adolescents may prefer to remain in a comfort zone that is logical, linguistic, left-brain, and cognitive-based processing. A bottom–up preferring clinician may struggle with this, especially if they note some needs related to bottom–up development, or somatic-held memories. Another child may struggle with Alexithymia and may not select their emotions in the way a clinician usually teaches within their modality. Again, this is where client self-determination is vital. It is important to recognize the child's needs, preferences, and preferred therapeutic approach. Once the modality is selected through collaboration between the neurodivergent client and therapist, it is important to be flexible and adaptive with the specific trauma-focused interventions.

## CASE EXAMPLE

Ana, a 16-year-old autistic female, was brought to therapy by her mother due to her aggressive behavior toward family members and struggles with dysregulation. Ana lived with her biological mother and two younger siblings. She was homeschooled and struggled with regulation, executive functioning issues (such as concentration and decision-making), and anxiety (primarily social anxiety). Ana's dysregulated state was described as a complete "shutdown." When this happened, she would become physically aggressive and attack her siblings. When Ana was in a state of regulation, she was well-spoken and artistic. She painted, created music, and sang. She spent much of her free time creating art. She had developed a social media presence and was hopeful that she would pursue a career in the arts.

AutPlay Therapy (a neurodiversity-affirming integrative play therapy framework) was implemented with Ana, as it is designed for autistic and other neurodivergent children. The Intake and Assessment Phase of AutPlay was implemented and focused on establishing relationship, discovering Ana's neurodivergent spectrum of presentation (which included her special interests and play preferences), and establishing therapy goals from an affirming perspective. At the completion of this therapy phase, it was established that one of Ana's therapies needs to be related to the trauma she was experiencing due to repeated social navigation struggles in a variety of settings resulting in rejection, embarrassment, anxiety, and dysregulation.

Addressing trauma in AutPlay Therapy requires a front-end process, which may lead to an integration of a traditional or specific trauma protocol. Before addressing trauma issues directly, the following three-step process was implemented with Ana:

Step 1 Relationship and safety—Neurodivergent children who have experienced trauma must begin with building a relationship with the therapist. With Ana, a non-directive philosophy was implemented with a focus on relationship development. The first few sessions were focused on discovering Ana's interests and allowing her to explore, ask questions, and become comfortable with the therapist and the therapy process.

Step 2 Regulation—Most neurodivergent children and adolescents will need to learn to regulate their systems. This can be done with a co-regulator or a regulation facilitator. AutPlay has three components to regulation—(a) Regulation Facilitator: Educating the child about their regulatory system and facilitating the process of regulation. (b) Co-Regulation: Being present and providing interactions that communicate being with and modeling regulating through dysregulated emotions and states. (c) Self-Regulation: The ability for the child to utilize, access, and implement a regulation process that they understand benefits their system. Several sessions were spent focusing on regulation with Ana. She progressed through the three components of AutPlay regulation and discovered various expressive art activities and processes that helped regulate her system. A "regulating lifestyle" was created with Ana. She had several art activities to choose from and would implement one per day for approximately 30–35 minutes. She would also implement regulating activities at other times as needed.

Step 3 Emotion recognition and expression—Autistic children may not understand, recognize, or express emotions in a neurotypical manner. In the case of Ana, it was discovered that she had Alexithymia, a condition where a person has difficulty identifying and expressing emotions. Ana had a difficult time using terms such as sad, anxious, and hurt to describe what she was feeling. Instead, she could identify states of being (feelings) by her energy level and through pictures and paintings that she created. Her ways of expressing emotions were understood and honored by the therapist and used during therapy.

After Ana had progressed through the AutPlay front-end process, it was determined that she could benefit from a more specific trauma protocol to address past trauma. The therapist decided to integrate EMDR protocol with AutPlay components and neurodiversity-affirming principles. As with many autistic and neurodivergent children, established trauma protocols such as EMDR can be effective and typically need to be altered to match the neurodivergent child's spectrum of presentation.

Ana struggled to engage in abstract cognitive processes. She could not create a safe place in her mind (visualization) or follow a guided relaxation. For a safe regulating space, Ana would listen to a music playlist on her phone while holding pulses for relaxation. This was done at the end of each session and anytime Ana needed regulation. It was difficult for Ana to maintain focus due to multitasking executive functioning issues (thinking about a memory, holding the pulses, noticing discomfort, and staying distracted from other thoughts or body sensations). During an EMDR set, the therapist would periodically give a verbal comment such as, "remember you are tracking a memory." It was difficult for Ana to stay regulated when processing a trauma memory. During an EMDR set, the therapist would periodically make a comment such as, "remember to take breaths" or "remember you are just watching your memory." These modifications allowed for a better fit between the EMDR process and Ana's neurodivergent presentation.

Ana's alexithymia required adjustment when checking in about feelings. Asking Ana to identify a feeling or using a traditional feeling chart was not effective. Both Ana and her therapist needed to conceptualize how she identified feelings and emotional states. It was discovered that Ana could identify feeling "normal," "calm," and "healthy energy," versus upset, overwhelmed, and "not right" through paintings and music. Several paintings and instrumental music compositions were selected that represented these various feelings and emotional states. During feeling check-ins and discussions, Ana would select the painting or piece of music for identification of what she was experiencing. The feelings, safe places, and executive functioning modifications were all necessary for Ana to experience the positive effects of the EMDR protocol.

Ana completed approximately 25 EMDR sessions. There were times the sessions paused to adjust or modify the protocol to best fit Ana. By the end of the 25 sessions, Ana's trauma-related symptoms seemed to be gone. She reported success in navigating social situations, feeling more confident about herself, and the ability to self-implement regulation tools whenever she felt she needed them. Overall, the integration of AutPlay processes and EMDR protocol with neurodiversity-affirming practices proved to be successful for Ana in addressing her trauma issues.

## CONCLUSION

The neurodivergent individual is often met with environments and systems that are both intentionally and unintentionally counter to the way their system understands and prefers to navigate. The result of this challenged navigation is a steady exposure to ableist experiences that communicate a lack of value and a constant bombardment of "you are different, and that is wrong." It is imperative that mental health therapists understand the neurodivergent experience, the real possibility of trauma needs, and neurodiversity-affirming practices to help address trauma and its co-occurring complexities.

## REFERENCES

Andersson, L. K. (2022). Autistic experiences of applied behavior analysis. *Autism: The International Journal of Research and Practice*, 8(23). https://doi.org/10.1177/13623613221118216

Beauchaine, T. P., Gatzke-Kopp, L., Neuhaus, E., Chipman, J., Reid, M. J., & Webster-Stratton, C. (2013). Sympathetic- and parasympathetic-linked cardiac function and prediction of externalizing behavior, emotion regulation, and prosocial behavior among preschoolers treated for ADHD. *Journal of Consulting and Clinical Psychology*, 81(3), 481–493.

Botha, M., & Gillespie-Lynch, K. (2022). Come as you are: Examining autistic identity development and the neurodiversity movement through an intersectional lens. *Human Development*, 66(2), 93–112.

Brown, N. M. (2022, November 7). Childhood trauma and ADHD: A complete overview & clinical guidance. *Additude*. https://www.additudemag.com/adhd-and-trauma-overview-signs-symptoms/

Brown, N. M., Brown, S. N., Briggs, R. D., Germán, M., Belamarich, P. F., & Oyeku, S. O. (2017, May–June). Associations between adverse childhood experiences and ADHD diagnosis and severity. *Academic Pediatrics*, *17*(4), 349–355. https://doi.org/10.1016/j.acap.2016.08.01

California Evidenced Based Clearinghouse for Child Welfare (2022, August 1). *Trauma treatment interventions*. https://www.cebc4cw.org/topic/trauma-treatment-client-level-interventions-child-adolescent/.

Cox, R. (2016). *The life recovery method: Autism treatment from a trauma perspective*. CreateSpace.

Dance, C. J., Ipser, A., & Simner, J. (2022). The prevalence of aphantasia (imagery weakness) in the general population. *Consciousness and Cognition*, *97*, 103243. https://doi.org/10.1016/j.concog.2021.103243

Eisenmenger, A. (2019, December 12). Ableism 101. *Access Living*. https://www.accessliving.org/newsroom/blog/ableism-101/

Fisher, N., Patel, H., van Diest, C., & Spain, D. (2022). Using eye movement desensitization and reprocessing (EMDR) with autistic individuals: A qualitative interview study with EMDR therapists. *Psychology and Psychotherapy*, *95*(4), 1071–1089.

Fuld, S. (2018). Autism spectrum disorder: The impact of stressful and traumatic life events and implications for clinical practice. *Clinical Social Work Journal*, *46*(3), 210–219.

Gajwani, R., & Minnis, H. (2023). Double jeopardy: Implications of neurodevelopmental conditions and adverse childhood experiences for child health. *European Child Adolescent Psychiatry*, *32*, 1–4. https://doi.org/10.1007/s00787-022-02081-9

Gates, G. (2019). *Trauma, stigma, and autism: Developing resilience and loosening the grip of shame*. Jessica Kingsley.

Grant, R. J. (2022). *Understanding sensory processing differences: A neurodiversity affirming guidebook for children and teens*. AutPlay Publishing.

Grant, R. J. (2023). *The AutPlay therapy handbook: Integrative family play therapy with neurodivergent children*. Routledge.

Guest, J. D., & Ohrt, J. H. (2018). Utilizing child centered play therapy with children diagnosed with autism spectrum disorder and enduring trauma: A case example. *International Journal of Play Therapy*, *27*(3), 157–165.

Haruvi-Lamdan, N., Horesh, D., Zohar, S., Kraus, M., & Golan, O. (2020). Autism spectrum disorder and post-traumatic stress disorder: An unexplored co-occurrence of conditions. *Autism: The International Journal of Research and practice*, *24*(4), 884–898.

Hoover, D. W. (2015). The effects of psychological trauma on children with autism spectrum disorders: A research review. *Journal of Autism and Developmental Disorders*, *2*(3), 287–299.

Hoover, D. W., & Kaufman, J. (2018). Adverse childhood experiences in children with autism spectrum disorder. *Current Opinion in Psychiatry*, *31*(2), 128–132.

Hurim, M., Sahin, S., & Kayihan, H. (2016). Evaluation of hand functions among children diagnosed with autism spectrum disorder with upper extremity trauma history. *Turkish Journal of Trauma and Emergency Surgery*, *22*(6), 559–565.

Im, D. S. (2016). Trauma as a contributor to violence in autism spectrum disorder. *Journal of Academic American Psychiatric Law, 44*(2), 184–192.

Kerns, C. M., Berkowitz, S. J., Moskowitz, L. J., Drahota, A., Lerner, M. D., Usual Care for Autism Study (UCAS) Consortium, & Newschaffer, C. J. (2020). Screening and treatment of trauma-related symptoms in youth with autism spectrum disorder among community providers in the United States. *Autism: The International Journal of Research and Practice, 24*(2), 515–525.

Kerns, C. M., Newschaffer, C. J., Berkowitz, S., & Lee, B. K. (2017). Brief report: Examining the association of autism and adverse childhood experiences in the national survey of children's health: The important role of income and co-occurring mental health conditions. *Journal of Autism and Developmental Disorders, 47*(7), 2275–2281.

Kirk, M. A., Taha, B., Dang, K., McCague, H., Hatzinakos, D., Katz, J., & Ritvo, P. (2022). A web-based cognitive behavioral therapy, mindfulness meditation, and yoga intervention for posttraumatic stress disorder: Single-arm experimental clinical trial. *JMIR Mental Health, 9*(2), e26479.

Lyons, S. (2019, September 1). *The repair of early trauma, a bottom-up approach.* Beacon House. https://beaconhouse.org.uk/wp-content/uploads/2019/09/Repair-of-Early-Trauma.pdf

Lowry, M. (n.d.). *Autistic trauma and internalized ableism.* Matt Lowry LPP. https://www.mattlowrylpp.com/blog/autistic-trauma-and-internalized-ableism.

Ryder, G. (2022, January 4). What is trauma? *PsychCentral.* https://psychcentral.com/health/what-is-trauma.

Reagan, L. (2021, October 22). *Trauma treatment modality series: "Top-down" and "bottom-up" approach to therapy.* Trauma Therapist Network. https://traumatherapistnetwork.com/trauma-treatment-modality-series-top-down-and-bottom-up-approach-to-therapy/

Robinson, A. (2018). Emotion focused therapy for autism spectrum disorder: A case conceptualization model for trauma related experiences. *Journal of Contemporary Psychotherapy, 48*(3), 133–143.

Spratt, E. G., Nicholas, J. S., Brady, K. T., Carpenter, L. A., Hatcher, C. R., Meekins, K. A., Furlanetto, R. W., & Charles, J. M. (2012). Enhanced cortisol response to stress in children in autism. *Journal of Autism and Developmental Disorders, 42*(1), 75–81.

Walker, N. (2021). *Neuroqueer heresies: Notes on the neurodiversity paradigm, autistic empowerment, and postnormal possibilities.* Autonomous Press.

Zackheim, L. (2007). Alexithymia: The expanding realm of research. *Journal of Psychosomatic Research, 63*(4), 345–347.

## CHAPTER TEN

# Exploring the Depths of BIPOC Experiences: The Repercussions of Individual and Collective Trauma

LILIANA BAYLON and JOSE TAPIA

This book chapter invites the reader to be curious and contemplate how individual and collective trauma can impact individuals and communities at large, particularly for Black, Indigenous, and People of Color (BIPOC). BIPOC is a widely used umbrella term specific to the United States and Canada when describing minoritized or racialized communities. As mental health therapists, we are aware of acute trauma (i.e., single trauma events), chronic trauma (i.e., repeated and prolonged events), and complex trauma (i.e., exposure to multiple traumatic events; invasive and interpersonal in nature). However, mental health therapists should be aware of other types of traumas when working with BIPOC individuals. BIPOC clients face historical trauma, intergenerational trauma, immigration trauma, cultural trauma, natural disaster trauma, terrorism trauma, pandemic trauma, and racial trauma.

Trauma is a direct personal experience of an event that involves actual or threatened death or serious injury, a threat to one's physical integrity, witnessing an event that involves the above experience, learning about unexpected or violent death, serious harm, or injury experienced by a family member or close associate (Lee & Boykins, 2022).

*Trauma Impacts: The Repercussions of Individual and Collective Trauma*, First Edition.
Edited by Jessica Stone, Robert J. Grant, and Clair Mellenthin.
© 2024 John Wiley & Sons, Inc. Published 2024 by John Wiley & Sons, Inc.

Historical trauma refers to an individual's cumulative experiences of emotional and psychological wounding, whereas intergenerational trauma is the historical trauma that spans multiple generations and affects communities and their descendants (Pumariega et al., 2022). Williams et al. (2017) shared that the combination of microaggressions, race-related stress, race-based traumatic events, and the school-to-prison pipeline has immense implications on the overall well-being of young people of color, as racism and discrimination are generally collective and cumulative traumas.

Immigration trauma is an accumulation of stressors, adjustments, and their cumulative effect as precipitants of the symptoms of distress. Aldana (2022) describes immigration trauma as psychological distress that includes four migration stages:

1. Premigration trauma (i.e., events experienced just before the migration that was a chief determinant of the relocation)
2. Traumatic events experienced during transit to the new country
3. Continuing traumatogenic experiences during the process of asylum-seeking and resettlement
4. Substandard living conditions in the host country due to unemployment, inadequate support, and minority persecution

Desjarlais et al. (1995) concluded that it is not migration alone but the traumatic or derailing events before, during, or after dislocation that lead to psychological distress of clinical proportions. Exposure to violence and other stressful life experiences of immigrant Latino families likely differs from those experienced by US-born Latinos. Among unaccompanied youth from Central America, premigration involves the sometimes-forced decision to migrate from war-related violence and drugs (Lustig et al., 2004). During migration, youth may be exposed to violence without familial support (Halvorsen, 2002). Postmigration, immigrant youth may have extended stays in detention centers, subsequent unstable living situations, and reunification with parents and family members who immigrated years before. In addition to these stressors, ongoing confrontations with acculturation challenges, daily stressors, and other types of traumatic events are related to poor mental health outcomes (Cleary et al., 2018).

Cultural trauma occurs when members of a collective group feel they have been subjected to a horrendous event that leaves indelible marks upon their group consciousness, marking their memories forever and changing their future identity in fundamental and irrevocable ways (Alexander et al., 2004). Table 10.1 provides a brief definition of trauma experiences.

**Table 10.1**
Definitions of Trauma Experiences

| Type of Trauma | Definition |
| --- | --- |
| Historical trauma | Cumulative emotional and psychological wounding, over the lifespan and across generations, emanates from massive group trauma experiences (Denham, 2008). |
| Intergenerational trauma | Refers to emotional and psychological wounding that is transmitted across generations (Cerdeña et al., 2021) |
| Immigration trauma | Also known as In-Transit Trauma, a person may experience trauma in relation to migration. Immigration trauma is thought of in different stages: Pre-migration trauma, Travel and transit, and Post-migration trauma (Aldana, 2022). |
| Cultural trauma | When members of a collectivity feel they have been subjected to a horrendous event that leaves indelible marks upon their group consciousness, marking their memories forever and changing their future identity in fundamental and irrevocable ways (Alexander et al., 2004). |
| Racial trauma | It deliberately targets persons of color because of their racial background (Jernigan & Daniel, 2011). |
| Individual trauma | Refers to the psychological and emotional harm experienced by an individual due to a single or a series of traumatic events (Ungar, 2013). |
| Collective trauma | Refers to the psychological and emotional harm experienced by a group due to a shared event or trauma experience (Raymond-Flesch et al., 2014). |

## HISTORY OF MALTREATMENT

In the United States, individuals who identify as BIPOC have endured decades of maltreatment, including, but not limited to slavery, segregation to racially biased laws and policies, disenfranchisement of voting rights, lack of representation in positions of power, inconsistent access to medical care, and unequal access to education. Additionally, individuals in these communities have experienced decades of domestic terror in the form of lynching, police brutality, the weaponization of the criminal justice system, forced removal from their lands, and the intentional dismantling of culturally relevant customs (Dunbar-Ortiz, 2014; Ortiz, 2018).

The history of systemic racism and discrimination has left a lasting impact on marginalized communities, creating a legacy of inequality and oppression. BIPOC individuals have endured generations of mistreatment that continue to shape their lived experiences today. The struggles faced by BIPOC communities encompass various aspects of life, including education, housing, employment, access to health care, and criminal justice. Disproportionate poverty rates, limited access to quality health care, and persistent racial profiling contribute to the ongoing marginalization of these individuals.

The consequences of this maltreatment are not only felt individually but also resonate throughout generations, as systemic barriers hinder progress and perpetuate cycles of disadvantage. These practices have continued with recent examples, such as the killing of unarmed Black men (Marisol Meraji & Demby, 2020), the separation of children from their families while seeking asylum at the border of Mexico (Carcamo, 2020), and the militarized attack on Indigenous individuals protecting their land at Standing Rock Indian Reservation (Estes & Dhillon, 2019).

## IMPACT OF COMPLEX TRAUMA ON BIPOC INDIVIDUALS AND COMMUNITIES

Complex trauma from a BIPOC perspective refers to the psychological and emotional effects of prolonged and repeated exposure to traumatic events and experiences explicitly faced by individuals in BIPOC communities (Cook et al., 2005). It encompasses the intersection of historical, intergenerational, and ongoing trauma resulting from systemic racism, discrimination, colonization, cultural erasure, and social injustice. Complex trauma recognizes that individuals from BIPOC backgrounds often face unique trauma due to systemic oppression, marginalization, and the historical legacy of colonization and slavery (Comas-Díaz et al., 2019). These traumas can have profound and long-lasting effects on individuals and communities, impacting their mental, emotional, and physical well-being. Complex trauma from a BIPOC perspective acknowledges that experiences of racism, microaggressions, xenophobia, institutionalized discrimination, and cultural disconnection can contribute to the development of complex post-traumatic stress disorder (PTSD) or other trauma-related disorders. These experiences can erode a person's sense of self, safety, trust, and belonging, leading to symptoms such as hypervigilance, emotional dysregulation, identity confusion, dissociation, depression, anxiety, and difficulties in interpersonal relationships.

In North American, European, and colonial zeitgeist societies, BIPOC experiences racial microaggressions, interpersonal, institutional, and systemic racism on a repetitive, constant, inevitable, and cumulative basis. Like complex trauma, racial trauma surrounds the victims' life course. It engenders consequences on their physical and mental health, behavior, cognition, relationships with others, self-concept, and social and economic life (Cénat, 2022). Although complex trauma differs from racial trauma in its origin, the consistency of racist victimization throughout the lifetime and the internalized racism associated with it create strong similarities in the experience and resulting complex symptomology (Cénat, 2022).

## RACE-BASED TRAUMATIC STRESS

Traditional research models (Lazarus & Folkman, 1984) studying the impact of stress posit that when an individual encounters a stimulus, that stimulus is appraised and deemed a stressor if the individual perceives the stimulus as unfavorable and if they do not have the internal resources to cope with it. Cultural models of stress (Clark et al., 1999; Harrell, 2000) expanded the traditional models by explicitly addressing racial and cultural factors from a social–political context that is more inclusive in evaluating stressful experiences of racial minority groups. Within this context, racial trauma refers to events of danger related to the real or perceived experience of racial discrimination, threats of harm and injury, and humiliating and shaming events, in addition to witnessing harm to other individuals because of actual or perceived racism (Lee & Boykins, 2022). In examining race-based traumatic stress, cultural stress models are necessary to center the experiences of BIPOC individuals encountering discrimination, oppression, and marginalization in their environment.

The American Psychiatric Association (2013) defined traumatic events as events that involve actual or threatened physical harm to oneself or others. This definition of traumatic events does not account for the range of experiences that can be encoded in an individual's body as trauma, especially for the BIPOC community. Racism has serious physical consequences on individuals, including hypertension, decreased heart rate variability, sleep difficulties, psychological distress, increased depression and anxiety, and other intense emotional experiences (Orejuela-Dávila, 2020). Due to these factors, racism is traumatic to the body, and the amount of race-based traumatic experiences will vary based on the individual's identities. A couple with the same racial and cultural identity will have unique experiences regarding race-based traumatic stress in the United States.

Race-based traumatic stress (Carter, 2007) is a conceptual framework that expands the cultural stress model to include traumatic experiences related to racist acts against BIPOC individuals. These events are considered psychological and emotional injuries that may contribute to or present themselves as mental health disorders (Orejuela-Dávila, 2020). Psychological injury implies that it is caused by external, situational, and environmental conditions, which impact an individual's view of self and others. There is frequently a violation of the person's core assumptions about the world and their human rights, putting the person in a state of extreme confusion and insecurity (Lee & Boykins, 2022). These conditions contribute to negative mental health outcomes.

## IDENTITY DEVELOPMENT AND INTERNALIZED RACISM

In exploring the impact of racism on BIPOC communities, it is essential to consider the psychological and emotional impact on individual's racial identity development. BIPOC encompasses various racial identities, and developmental theories reflect both singular racial identities and multiracial/biracial/mixed-race identity development. Racial identity development theories are not meant as prescriptive states of an individual's journey toward an self-understanding. Rather, they serve as a framework to understand the various ways individuals navigate their own understanding of held racial identities within the context of the United States. The following racial identity development theories reflect some common frameworks, but many more exist that this section will not mention.

For Black-identifying individuals, Cross and Fhagen-Smith (2001) described a six-sector framework of racial identity development that describes their conceptualization of becoming Black: (a) infancy and childhood in early Black identity development, (b) preadolescence, (c) adolescence, (d) early adulthood, (e) adult nigrescence, and (f) nigrescence recycling. Cross (1991) defined nigrescence as the process of becoming Black and developing a racial identity. During preadolescence, internalized racism may develop based on the individual's lived experiences during crucial developmental periods. If internalized racism is not addressed over time, individuals may disown their Blackness. An individual who achieves nigrescence recycling has an integrated self-concept that is positive.

Latinx identity development, as described by Ferdman and Gallegos (2001), provides six orientations focused on ways Latines come to think about themselves in a diverse and ever-changing society, against the backdrop of a range of historical and cultural influences: (a) white-identified, (b) undifferentiated/denied, (c) Latino as other, (d) subgroup-identified, (e) Latino-identified, and (f) Latino-integrated. These are the six orientations that Ferdman and Gallegos (2001) describe as a process rather than stages of development. Many racial identity development models describe the process beginning with a white-centered narrative and moving into their own racial identity development.

Kim's (2012) Asian American Identity Development Model emphasizes six stages of racial identity to highlight the social and psychological consequences of being racially minoritized in the United States: (a) ethical awareness, (b) white identification, (c) awakening to social–political consciousness, (d) redirection to Asian American consciousness, and (e) incorporation. These sequential and progressive stages provide a framework for the process an Asian American individual navigates as they develop their own racial identity.

Since many Americans are not born with one racial identity, identity development theories also consider biracial individuals to expand our understanding of experiencing the world with more than one racial identity. The Continuum of Biracial Identity Model (Rockquemore & Laszloffy, 2005) attempts to reflect the diverse ways multiracial individuals see themselves racially, without judging them if they do not see themselves as the models suggest. While these identity developmental models are frameworks to aid in conceptualization, it is essential that the therapist's focus be on the client as the expert in their experience.

## SYSTEMIC IMPACT OF TRAUMA

Individual trauma refers to the psychological and emotional harm experienced by an individual due to a single or a series of traumatic events. For example, traumatic experiences include physical or emotional abuse, natural disasters, accidents, and violent crimes. On the other hand, collective trauma refers to the psychological and emotional harm experienced by a group due to a shared event or trauma experience. Examples of collective trauma experiences can include war (e.g., Ukraine and Drug Cartel), terrorism (e.g., September 11), natural disasters (e.g., hurricanes, fires, tsunamis, and earthquakes), and social injustice (e.g., Sandy Hook, racial killings, restriction of human rights, gun violence, separation of families, and children in cages). One of the key differences between individual and collective trauma is that collective trauma affects a group of people rather than just one individual. As a result, collective trauma can be felt on a larger scale and can significantly affect communities, societies, and even entire cultures (e.g., pandemics and recessions).

Another essential difference between individual and collective trauma is how they are experienced and processed. Individual trauma is often processed on a personal level, with individuals experiencing fear, anger, and helplessness (Downing, 2007; Hirschberger, 2018; Paliewicz & Hasian, 2016). Conversely, collective trauma is often processed on a communal level, with the affected group experiencing shared grief and loss (e.g., the COVID-19 global pandemic, Sandy Hook, where a mass shooting took the lives of multiple children in an elementary school, and the 2019 Texas Walmart shooting, another mass shooting in which the shooter purposefully shot and killed Latine individuals). Both individual and collective trauma can have significant long-term effects on the individuals and communities affected by them, including feelings of helplessness, anxiety, depression, and PTSD. Therefore, acknowledging and addressing both types of traumas are essential to promote healing for those impacted.

Pumariega et al. (2022) revealed that traumatic experiences disproportionately affect minority youth. These experiences include historical/generational trauma, immigration, acculturation stressors, natural and man-made disasters, experiences of discrimination, family violence, and community violence. Despite the higher incidence of trauma exposure, minority youth are less likely to access medical and mental health care. These disparities result in increased rates of depression, anxiety, post-traumatic stress, substance use disorders, and suicide in minority youth (Pumariega et al., 2022).

Although trauma research has arisen largely from an individual psychotherapeutic paradigm, there is growing awareness that traumatic events resulting from war, intercommunal conflicts, and other forms of collective violence impact societies at large. Existing literature has established the notion of collective trauma to characterize how traumatic events such as legal attacks, violence, disasters, and racism can have lasting impacts on communities (Alexander et al., 2004). An example of collective trauma worldwide is the global COVID-19 pandemic. The world was paralyzed, and had a shared feeling of uncertainty, helplessness, fear, and anger. Collective trauma can be felt and seen in racial trauma (e.g., anti-Black racial violence, children in cages, children separated from their parents, and community shootings), gender trauma (e.g., LGBTQIA+ communities and women's rights), and hate crimes (e.g., race, religion, and gender).

In their research, Raymond-Flesch et al. (2014) state that Latinos, like other ethnic and cultural groups, have experienced collective trauma. Examples of Latino collective trauma include colonization, unfavorable government policies (e.g., the Deferred Action for Childhood Arrivals [DACA] program, family separation at the U.S.–Mexico border, detention in immigration facilities, and deportation), and immigration-related trauma (e.g., discrimination, racial bias, and negative stereotypes).

Trauma can significantly impact individuals, families, and even larger systemic structures (collective trauma). Trauma can impact an individual's emotional, psychological, and physical well-being. As mentioned throughout the chapter, it can lead to mental health issues such as PTSD, depression, anxiety, and other mental health issues. Trauma can also impact an individual's ability to form healthy relationships, cope with stress, and function in daily life.

Trauma can also impact larger systemic structures, such as communities. Trauma can perpetuate cycles of violence and oppression, which can have long-lasting impacts on the affected communities. It can also lead to systemic issues such as lack of access to resources, poverty, and homelessness. Therefore, it is essential to recognize the impact of trauma on all levels and work toward prevention and healing at each level. As mental health therapists, this may involve offering individual therapy, family therapy, community-based interventions, and advocating for systemic changes to address the root causes of trauma.

## Impact on Family System

Traumatic experiences impact the entire family system. Family members may experience similar symptoms as the primary victim, such as anxiety and depression. They may also experience relational difficulties due to the impact of trauma on the family dynamic. For example, family members may struggle with communication, trust, and emotional regulation. Chronic experiences of stress due to race-based traumatic stress correlate to negative health outcomes (i.e., high blood pressure, diabetes, and chronic illnesses) for all ages, not only adults within a family system (Brody et al., 2014). Considerations for how everyone within a BIPOC family experiences trauma through a developmental lens provide an opportunity to view the system more accurately (Daniels, 2022). The presentation of the family systems responding to trauma will vary based on their individually held identities and their lived experiences. Lastly, framing the family's behavior as a response to trauma instead of "bad" or "maladaptive" provides an opportunity for validating the race-based stress being experienced (Daniels, 2022).

## Intergenerational Trauma

Intergenerational or transgenerational trauma refers to emotional and psychological wounding transmitted across generations. For example, Latinx individuals who have migrated from Latin America to the United States or Canada and their descendants have been vulnerable to intergenerational trauma due to legacies of colonialism, political violence, and migration-related stressors (Cerdeña et al., 2021). Intergenerational trauma refers to the transmission of trauma from parent figures to their infants or children, resulting in the effects of trauma experienced by the second generation without exposure to the original traumatic experience or event (Hesse & Main, 2000). Intergenerational trauma occurs when parent figures who have experienced trauma transmit the effects of their trauma to their children via interactional patterns, genetic pathways, and/or family dynamics (Hesse & Main, 2000). Learning to think and behave in ways that replicate their caregivers' traumatic adaptations or by being exposed to the secondary psychosocial effects of these adaptations and themselves similarly having to adapt (O'Neill et al., 2018; Weiss & Weiss, 2000). Transmission occurs unintentionally and usually without awareness of the contribution of the original traumatic event (O'Neill et al., 2018).

## Impact on Community

Trauma can also impact larger systemic structures, such as communities. Trauma can perpetuate cycles of violence and oppression, which can have long-lasting impacts on the affected communities. It can also lead to systemic issues such as lack of access to resources, poverty, and homelessness. Therefore, it is essential to recognize the impact of trauma on all levels and work toward prevention and healing at each level. As mental health therapists, this may involve offering individual therapy, family therapy, community-based interventions, and advocating for systemic changes to address the root causes of trauma.

## Sociocultural Factors

How BIPOC clients interpret and respond to a traumatic experience is embedded in various sociocultural factors. Some of these factors include gender, socioeconomic status, cultural background, mental health history, age, housing situation, and sexual orientation, among many others (Blueford & Adams, 2021). BIPOC communities face higher rates of psychosocial disparities such as poverty, lack of education, and barriers to health and mental health services. In addition, exposure to multiple stressors such as discrimination, racism, community violence exposure, and immigration and acculturation stresses increases traumatic stress. These composite stressors increase mental health morbidity rates, such as depression, suicidality, stress-related disorders, school disciplinary actions, incarceration, and placement in state custody (Pumariega et al., 2022).

## Racism

Racism is defined as a system of racial group designations based on dominance, whereby the majority view minority groups as inferior and are oppressed at individual, institutional, and cultural levels (Harrell, 2000). Racial trauma refers to experiences related to threats, prejudices, harm, shame, humiliation, and guilt associated with various types of racial discrimination, either for direct victims or witnesses (Comas-Díaz, 2016; Helms et al., 2010).

The United States has undergone a significant increase in non-European populations over the past 50 years. This has been both a result of demographic changes (i.e., aging of the non-Hispanic White/European origin populations); greater growth of African American, Latinx, Asian origin, and American Indian populations; and significant immigration from Latin America, Southeast and East Asia, the Middle East, and Africa. As of 2020, most children and youth in the United States are from these minority, non-European backgrounds (this will be the case for the overall population by 2045; Pumariega et al., 2022). Due to the inequities mentioned above, these populations face higher rates of psychosocial disparities such as poverty, lack of education, barriers to health and mental health services, and exposure to multiple stressors such as discrimination, racism, community violence exposure, and immigration and acculturation stresses. These composite stressors increase mental health morbidity rates, such as depression, suicidality, stress-related disorders, school disciplinary actions, incarceration, placement in state custody, and trauma-related issues.

## FUTURE PROJECTIONS, CONCERNS, AND SUGGESTIONS

Based on current events and concerns mentioned throughout the book chapter, it is possible to make some projections and identify potential concerns regarding individual and collective trauma in the United States or worldwide. However, one concern is the ongoing COVID-19 pandemic, which has already caused significant individual and collective trauma in the United States and worldwide. The pandemic has disrupted daily life and led to widespread illness, death, and economic hardship. The long-term mental health consequences of the pandemic, such as increased rates of anxiety, depression, and PTSD, are still unclear but are likely to be significant.

Another concern is the ongoing political polarization and social unrest in the United States, amplified by social media. The Black Lives Matter protests, immigrant detentions, separation of families at the border, children in cages, LGBTQI+ discrimination, reproductive rights, and the storming of the U.S. Capitol have all contributed to collective trauma and instability in the country. Climate change (e.g., hurricanes, wildfires, and floods) and man-made disasters, such as mass shootings, can also contribute to individual and collective trauma. Individuals, communities, and policymakers must prioritize mental health and trauma-informed care to address these concerns.

## CONCLUSION

Individual and collective trauma has been significant for BIPOC communities. These traumas result from systemic racism, discrimination, and violence experienced by BIPOC individuals and communities in the United States and Canada. BIPOC individuals face their own personal experiences of trauma and the collective trauma passed down through generations. The impact of this trauma on the mental, physical, and emotional well-being of BIPOC individuals cannot be overstated. It can lead to feelings of helplessness, anger, anxiety, and depression. It can also contribute to physical health problems, such as chronic pain, fatigue, and insomnia. However, there is hope. The BIPOC community has a long history of resilience, strength, and resistance. Healing from trauma is a long process, but it is possible with the help of support systems. Community support, culturally sensitive therapists, and self-care practices can all be practical tools for healing. By acknowledging the impact of individual and collective trauma and supporting each other in the healing process, we can create an equitable society for all.

In clinical work, it is important to consider and explore the clients' identities in counseling. Providing space to broach with clients about their held identities allows them to begin creating a therapeutic environment that allows for identity exploration. During these crucial conversations early and throughout therapy, the client can discuss difficult experiences related to racism, discrimination, and marginalization. The therapist can begin to conceptualize the depth of internalized racism and psychological trauma experienced by the client.

## REFERENCES

Aldana, R. E. (2022). Taming immigration trauma. *Cardozo Law Review, 44*(2), 387–476.

Alexander, J. C., Eyeman, R., Giensen, B., Smelser, N. J., & Sztompka, P. (2004). Toward a theory of cultural trauma. In *Cultural trauma and collective identity* (1st ed., pp. 1–30). University of California Press. http://www.jstor.org/stable/10.1525/j.ctt1pp9nb.4

Blueford, J. M., & Adams, C. R. (2021). Trauma-informed grief counseling with older BIPOC individuals. *Adultspan Journal, 20*(2), 111–124. https://doi.org/10.1002/adsp.12114

Brody, G. H., Simons, R. L., Chae, D. H., Yu, T., Kogan, S. M., & Beach, S. R. H. (2014). Perceived discrimination among African American adolescents and allostatic load: A longitudinal analysis with buffering effects. *Child Development, 85*(3), 989–1002. https://doi.org/10.1111/cdev.12213

Carcamo, C. (2020, October 24). Parents of 545 children separated at the U.S.-Mexico border have not been located [Interview]. In *Weekend Edition Saturday*. NPR. https://www.npr.org/2020/10/24/927384388/parents-of-545-children-separated-at-u-s-mexico-border-have-not-been-located

Carter, R. T. (2007). Racism and psychological and emotional injury. *The Counseling Psychologist, 35*(1), 13–105. https://doi.org/10.1177/0011000006292033

Cénat, J. M. (2022). Complex racial trauma: Evidence, theory, assessment, and treatment. *Perspectives on Psychological Science*, 174569162211204. https://doi.org/10.1177/17456916221120428

Cerdeña, J. P., Rivera, L. M., & Judy, M. (2021). Intergenerational trauma in Latinxs: A scoping review. *Social Science & Medicine, 270*, 113662. https://doi.org/10.1016/j.socscimed.2020.113662

Clark, R., Anderson, N. H., Clark, V. R., & Williams, D. R. (1999). Racism as a stressor for African Americans: A biopsychosocial model. *American Psychologist, 54*(10), 805–816. https://doi.org/10.1037/0003-066x.54.10.805

Cleary, S. P., Snead, R., Dietz-Chavez, D., Rivera, I., & Edberg, M. (2018). Immigrant trauma and mental health outcomes among Latino youth. *Journal of Immigrant and Minority Health, 20*(5), 1053–1059. https://doi.org/10.1007/s10903-017-0673-6

Comas-Díaz, L. (2016). Racial trauma recovery: A race-informed therapeutic approach to racial wounds. In *American Psychological Association eBooks* (pp. 249–272). https://doi.org/10.1037/14852-012

Comas-Díaz, L., Hall, G. C. N., & Neville, H. J. (2019). Racial trauma: Theory, research, and healing: Introduction to the special issue. *American Psychologist, 74*(1), 1–5. https://doi.org/10.1037/amp0000442

Cook, A., Spinazzola, J., Ford, J., Lanktree, C., Blaustein, M., Cloitre, M., DeRosa, R., Hubbad, R., Kagan, R., Liautaud, J., Mallah, K., Olafson, E., & van der Kolk, B. (2005). Complex trauma in children and adolescents. *Psychiatric Annals, 35*(5), 390–398.

Cross, W. E., Jr. (1991). *Shades of Black: Diversity in African American identity.* Temple University Press.

Cross, W. E., Jr., & Fhagen-Smith, P. E. (2001). Patterns of African American identity development: A life span perspective. In C. L. Wijeyesinghe & B. W. Jackson (Eds.), *New perspectives on racial identity development: A theoretical and practical anthology* (pp. 243–270). New York University Press.

Daniels, A. D. (2022). Combining family systems approaches to address BIPOC families' racial trauma amidst the global pandemic. *The Family Journal, 30*(2), 157–163. https://doi.org/10.1177/10664807221078969

Denham, A. R. (2008). Rethinking historical trauma: Narratives of resilience. *Transcultural Psychiatry, 45*(3), 391–414.

Desjarlais, R., Eisenberg, L., Good, B., & Kleinman, A. (1995). *World mental health.* Oxford University Press.

Downing, J. R. (2007). No greater sacrifice: American airlines employee crisis response to the September 11 attack. *Journal of Applied Communication Research, 35*(4), 350–375. https://doi.org/10.1080/00909880701611078

Dunbar-Ortiz, R. (2014). *An Indigenous Peoples' history of the United States.* Beacon Press.

Estes, D., & Dhillon, J. (2019). *Standing with standing rock: Voices from the #NoDAPL movement.* University of Minnesota Press.

Ferdman, B. M., & Gallegos, P. I. (2001). Racial identity development and Latinos in the United States. In C. L. Wijeyesinghe & B. W. Jackson, III (Eds.), *New perspectives on racial identity development: A theoretical and practical anthology* (pp. 32–66). University Press.

Halvorsen, K. (2002). Separated children seeking asylum, the most vulnerable of all. *Forced Migration Review, 12,* 34–36.

Harrell, S. P. (2000). A multidimensional conceptualization of racism-related stress: Implications for the well-being of people of color. *American Journal of Orthopsychiatry, 70*(1), 42–57. https://doi.org/10.1037/h0087722

Helms, J. E., Nicolas, G., & Green, C. E. (2010). Racism and ethnoviolence as trauma: Enhancing professional training. *Traumatology, 16*(4), 53–62. https://doi.org/10.1177/1534765610389595

Hesse, E., & Main, M. (2000). Disorganization in infant and adult attachment: Description, correlates, and implications for developmental psychopathology. *Journal of the American Psychoanalytic Association, 48*(4), 1097–1127.

Hirschberger, G. (2018). Collective trauma and the social construction of meaning. *Frontiers in Psychology, 9.* https://doi.org/10.3389/fpsyg.2018.01441

Jernigan, M. M., & Daniel, J. H. (2011). Racial trauma in the lives of Black Children and Adolescents: Challenges and clinical implications. *Journal of Child & Adolescent Trauma, 4*(2), 123–141. https://doi.org/10.1080/19361521.2011.574678

Kim, J. (2012). Asian American identity development theory. In C. L. Wijeyesinghe & B. W. Jackson, III (Eds.), *New perspectives on racial identity development: A theoretical and practical anthology* (pp. 67–90). University Press.

Lazarus, R. S., & Folkman, S. (1984). *Stress, appraisal and coping*. Springer.

Lee, C. C., & Boykins, M. (2022). Racism as a mental health challenge: An antiracist counseling perspective. *Canadian Psychology, 63*(4), 471–478. https://doi.org/10.1037/cap0000350

Lustig, S. L., Kia-Keating, M., Knight, W. G., Geltman, P., Ellis, H., Kinzie, J. D., et al. (2004). Review of child and adolescent refugee mental health. *Journal of the American Academy of Child and Adolescent Psychiatry, 43*, 24–36. [PubMed: 14691358]

Marisol Meraji, S., & Demby, G. (Hosts). (2020, May 3). A decade of watching Black people die [Audio podcast episode]. *In Code Switch*. NPR. https://www.npr.org/2020/05/29/865261916/a-decade-ofwatching-black-people-die

O'Neill, L., Fraser, T., Kitchenham, A., & McDonald, V. (2018). Hidden burdens: A review of intergenerational, historical and complex trauma, implications for indigenous families. *Journal of Child & Adolescent Trauma, 11*(2), 173–186.

Orejuela-Dávila, A. I. (2020). Posttraumatic growth and race-based trauma among African Americans [Unpublished doctoral dissertation]. The University of North Carolina at Charlotte.

Ortiz, P. (2018). *An African American and Latinx history of the United States*. Beacon Press.

Paliewicz, N. S., & Hasian, M. (2016). Mourning absences, melancholic commemoration, and the contested public memories of the national September 11 memorial and museum. *Western Journal of Communication, 80*(2), 140–162. https://doi.org/10.1080/10570314.2015.1128559

Pumariega, A. J., Jo, Y., Beck, B., & Rahmani, M. (2022). Trauma and US minority children and youth. *Current Psychiatry Reports, 24*(4), 285–295. https://doi.org/10.1007/s11920-022-01336-1

Raymond-Flesch, M., Siemons, R., Pourat, N., Jacobs, K., & Brindis, C. D. (2014). "There is no help out there, and if there is, it's really hard to find": A qualitative study of the health concerns and health care access of Latino "DREAMers". *Journal of Adolescent Health, 55*(3), 323–328.

Rockquemore, K. A., & Laszloffy, T. A. (2005). *Moving beyond tragedy: A multidimensional model of Mixed-Race identity. Raising Biracial Children*. http://ci.nii.ac.jp/ncid/BA90576298

Ungar, M. (2013). Resilience, trauma, context, and culture. *Trauma, Violence & Abuse, 14*(3), 255–266. https://doi.org/10.1177/1524838013487805

Weiss, M., & Weiss, S. (2000). Second generation to holocaust survivors. *American Journal of Psychotherapy, 54*(3), 372–385. https://doi.org/10.1176/appi.psychotherapy.2000.54.3.372

Williams, M. T., Negrón, A. P. P., & Mier-Chairez, J. (2017). Tools for assessing racism-related stress and trauma among Latinos. In *Springer eBooks* (pp. 71–95). https://doi.org/10.1007/978-3-319-64880-4_4

## CHAPTER ELEVEN

# Working with Refugees: Creating Connection and Therapeutic Refuge

ANNE STEWART, JULIA LINGER, JENNIFER NELSON FAULCONER,
and HANNAH JARRETT

## DEFINITION AND OVERVIEW OF REFUGEE STATUS

Over 100 million people worldwide, the highest number on record and 1% of the global population, have been forcibly displaced from their homes due to violence or persecution. Of this total, over 32 million qualify as refugees, half of whom are children (United Nations High Commissioner for Refugees [UNHCR], 2023). A refugee is a person who has fled their home country due to persecution, war, or violence, crossed international borders in search of safety, and who has been recognized by United Nations conventions as in need of protection (UNHCR, 2023). "Refugee" is a legal term that is widely misunderstood and often politicized.[1] Five million are asylum seekers who hope for international protection but whose claims for refugee status have

---

[1] A refugee is defined as a person who "owing to a well-founded fear of being persecuted for reasons of race, religion, nationality, membership of a particular social group, or political opinion, is outside the country of his nationality, and is unable to or, owing to such fear, is unwilling to avail himself of the protection of that country" (UNHCR, 2010, p. 14). The chapter will use this definition of refugee.

*Trauma Impacts: The Repercussions of Individual and Collective Trauma*, First Edition.
Edited by Jessica Stone, Robert J. Grant, and Clair Mellenthin.
© 2024 John Wiley & Sons, Inc. Published 2024 by John Wiley & Sons, Inc.

not yet been accepted. Many others are either migrants,[2] who have left their home country not for asylum-seeking, or internally displaced persons (IDP), who have been forced to flee their homes, but did not cross an international border. IDPs are neither legally protected by international law nor eligible for many types of aid because they are legally under the protection of their own government (UNHCR, 2023). Man-made circumstances such as severe economic hardship, widespread violations of human rights, and other manifestations, which seriously disturb the public order as well as natural or ecological disasters, are not currently recognized. The distinctions among asylum seekers, migrants, IDPs, and refugee status are more complex and nuanced than they might first seem, and each of us encounters the refugee crisis in a deeply personal way that intersects with our own professional and personal beliefs and values. As you read the chapter, we encourage you to reflect and imagine how the information impacts the vulnerable and resilient population displaced from their homes.

## PSYCHOLOGICAL IMPACT OF TRAUMA ON REFUGEES

The refugee experience is often understood according to the stages of premigration, migration, and postmigration.

### PREMIGRATION

During the premigration stage, refugees may experience violence, war, sexual abuse, slavery, torture, and/or prolonged detention. They often feel anxiety about the conditions in their country, fear of persecution, and anticipated sadness about their losses (Gwozdziewycs & Mehl-Madrona, 2013). Many refugees may have experienced a "disappearance" of a family member or a forced abduction as an act of violence due to religious, political, or ethnic conflict. These are key tools of civil wars, state repression, and terrorism, and lead to collective and intergenerational trauma. At the individual level, refugees may experience depression, grief, hypervigilance, and prolonged states of anxiety, sleep disorders, fear, anger, and guilt (Carll et al., 2021). At the family level, they may experience stressors unique to ambiguous loss, disruptions in economic well-being, and feelings of powerlessness. The extreme nature of these traumas makes refugees particularly susceptible to traumatic stress disorders and prolonged neurobiological alterations in their stress response system.

---

[2] "Migrant" is not defined under international law. The United Nations International Organization for Migration (2023) defines a migrant as "a person who moves away from his or her place of usual residence, whether within a country or across an international border, temporarily or permanently, and for a variety of reasons." Migrant circumstances can also be characterized as "voluntary" or "forced" migration.

## MIGRATION

The migration stage may be discrete or prolonged, depending on the time it takes refugees to escape their home country and whether they go to a refugee camp. Those placed in refugee camps often remain for many years (UNHCR, 2023). The stressors experienced during this stage may include exposure to frightening and life-threatening conditions, such as ethnic and gender-based violence, detention, hunger, vulnerability to human trafficking, and lack of access to services to cover their basic needs (Carll et al., 2021). These stressors are cumulative, adding to the trauma experienced during the premigration stage. Because there is no opportunity to process the psychological reactions generated during the premigration phase, the refugee's levels of distress, anxiety, fear, grief, and depression are likely to continue and compound (Nosè et al., 2017).

## POSTMIGRATION

The postmigration stage includes both short-term and long-term adjustment. During the initial transition period, refugees may experience a wide range of emotions, including depression, fear of the unknown, helplessness or hopelessness, survivor's guilt, or anger. The laws, economic and political stability, and resources of the country to which they escape will greatly impact refugees' well-being. Two out of every three refugees endure a "protracted refugee" experience, defined as 5 or more years exiled from their home country (Hilado et al., 2021). As refugees adjust to their new location, they may mourn the loss of family, friends, and familiar culture. Family separation is a tremendous source of distress and may contribute to increased symptoms of depression and anxiety. Refugees may also experience discrimination, concerns for their economic survival, and fear of deportation (Nosé et al., 2017).

# CURRENT MANIFESTATIONS FOR WORKING WITH REFUGEES

When working with refugees, it is imperative to adopt an ecological or contextual orientation in your work to acknowledge and understand the additive effects of trauma. In this section, research findings that help guide treatment at the individual, family, and community levels are explored.

## CONTEXTUAL CONSIDERATIONS

Addressing basic needs for safety and food can help restore a sense of safety and control (Carll et al., 2021). Consider what role you might serve in overcoming common barriers to care, such as lack of access to affordable housing and transportation, the need for knowledge about available services, and poor coordination between hospitals and community-based services. Addressing basic needs for safety and food can help restore a sense of safety and control (Carll et al., 2021). Clinicians can promote and help coordinate access to education, and physical, mental, and social care to foster a sense of belonging and connection. Because poor social integration is associated with higher rates of anxiety and depression, clinicians also need to be knowledgeable about programs that promote social integration, such as language classes, vocational training, and peer mentorship programs. In addition, the use of interpreters can aid in culturally responsive rapport building, engaging with treatment, and obtaining a job (Carll et al., 2021).

## Relevant Issues

Refugees create ways to function and reimagine their lives while experiencing repeated periods of transition, stress, and uncertainty. While these transitional periods can foment feelings of disequilibrium and forced adjustment, clinicians and service providers are invited to view the refugee experience through a strengths-based lens of resilience and hope. Generating processes that ensure refugees' voice and agency within the context of their transition helps to broaden the scope of healing beyond the trauma and into a sense of "being, belonging, and becoming" (Vindevogel & Verelst, 2020, p. 55).

Approaching your engagement with a deep sense of cultural humility is essential for working with refugee individuals and families. Cultural humility includes a commitment to lifelong self-evaluation/reflection, redressing systemic power imbalances, and developing and maintaining respectful relationships based on mutual trust (Murray-Garcia & Tervalon, 2017). Cultural humility allows for an openness to options in therapeutic approaches and the scope of the provider's role. Community connections are strengthened by acknowledging and welcoming collective worldviews and cultural diversities, in contrast to the more individualistic Western therapeutic models that champion independent individual functioning over interdependence. Increasing awareness of cultural, sociopolitical, and social justice components of the refugee experience is vital for avoiding "psychological colonialism" (Bemak & Chung, 2021). The use of cultural brokers and interpreters as part of the interprofessional community care team can help to bridge gaps in understanding based on language and culture (Frounfelker et al., 2020). Positioning oneself solidly into a cultural humility framework cultivates a space to bear witness to refugee migratory grief and personal narratives, and to provide compassionate, empathic, and validating responses.

A meaningful concept is the idea of "place attachment," or the bond that develops between a person and place, especially related to the resettlement process. Providers may assist refugees in exploring ways to honor emotional ties to their former homes while finding support to nurture bonds in their new place, highlighting the value of a sense of continuity (Albers et al., 2021). A large-scale, population-based cohort study of refugees aged from birth to 16 years, conducted by Foverskov et al. (2022), found that higher neighborhood disadvantage was associated with an increased risk of psychiatric disorders before the age of 30. This study offers another perspective for considering the impact of "place" and the targeted settlement of refugee families in less disadvantaged areas to enhance the long-term mental health of refugee children and adolescents.

While not all refugees will develop problematic symptoms, refugees have left their home countries because of threats to their lives or freedom and are, understandably, more likely than the general population to have experienced traumatic events (Nosé et al., 2017). As with most research findings, there is a correlation between the severity of trauma experienced and the severity of symptoms. In addition to working from a contextual framework, it is vital to balance evidence-based treatment approaches with culturally and linguistically congruent healing traditions and beliefs. Trauma-informed care is a relevant treatment framework to use with refugees that involves understanding, recognizing, and responding to all types of traumas. This approach emphasizes physical, psychological, and emotional safety for both clients and providers, and helps survivors rebuild a sense of control and empowerment. Trauma-informed care acknowledges the profound disruptive impact of traumatic experiences on physiological regulation and the corresponding need for bottom–up interventions. Importantly, trauma-informed care also refers to an organizational structure and promotes processes that recognize the pervasive influence of trauma (Substance Abuse and Mental Health Services Administration, 2014).

## INTERVENTIONS FOR WORKING WITH REFUGEES

A number of approaches have been found to positively address the disruptive impact of traumatic events experienced by refugees. Recommended trauma treatments incorporate findings from neuroscience and emphasize the importance of implementing sensory-based and motor interventions within the context of a strong and positive therapeutic relationship. For many refugees, prolonged activation of their stress response systems may make them particularly vulnerable to threats, fixed in a state of sympathetic activation and feelings of anxiety, panic, or irritation. Others may be caught in a state of dorsal vagal activation, feeling dissociated, numb, or hopeless (Porges, 2011). Perry (2006) named six core characteristics of therapeutic experiences that serve as a guide for creating trauma-informed interventions. The dimensions are relational, relevant, repetitive, rewarding, rhythmic, and respectful. In addition, holistic, multimodal, and community-based interventions, which enable refugees to have reparative experiences and trusting relationships, need to be front and center for service providers.

## Narrative Approaches

Narrative therapeutic approaches have been found to be effective in working with traumatized refugee populations (Lely et al., 2019). Researchers and providers have noted the need to bridge the gap between a refugee individual's lived experience of trauma during the migration process and a productive path toward emotional and neurobiological healing (O'Brien & Charura, 2022). Narrative exposure therapy (Lely et al., 2019) can provide a framework for making meaning and help those managing trauma and post-traumatic stress disorder (PTSD) to restructure memories and integrate contradictory events. Umer and Elliot (2018) used narrative writing exercises with refugees in the post-migration phase in order to study hope, and ultimately, post-traumatic growth, as integral protective factors for healing.

## Storytelling

Storytelling can help children share their thoughts and make sense of their world, and can also engage families, teachers, and communities in discussion. KIDNET adapts narrative therapy for children through play by incorporating familiar objects and toys. For example, a string could signify a child's life, with rocks or drawings placed along it that may signify traumatic events, and flowers could represent hopes and dreams for the future (Gwozdziewycs & Mehl-Madrona, 2013). Books with salient themes can help give words and normalize experiences such as leaving home and mourning a loss of language and culture. Both books and oral storytelling can help children express and explore their experiences, in the same way that narrative therapy does with adults.

## Trauma-Focused Cognitive Behavioral Therapy

Trauma-focused cognitive behavioral therapy (TF-CBT) is an evidence-based intervention demonstrated to be effective across the lifespan for addressing a variety of behavioral and emotional problems. TF-CBT is short-term, structured, and skill-based.

Practitioners using TF-CBT with children and their caregivers teach PRACTICE skills (Psychoeducation, Relaxation, Affective Modulation, Cognitive Coping, Trauma Narrative and Emotional Processing, In vivo Desensitization, Conjoint Session, and Enhancing Safety; Unterhitzenberger et al., 2015), which have been shown to significantly reduce both internalizing and externalizing symptoms after a traumatic event. Unterhitzenberger et al. (2015) successfully adapted the PRACTICE process to the needs of an 18-year-old adolescent male client, with refugee status, by modifying *P-Psychoeducation* to include psychoeducation about dissociation, increasing *R-Relaxation* over multiple sessions, and naming feelings in both languages for *A-Affective.*

## Experiential Activities and Expressive Arts

Providers can offer opportunities to engage experientially through creative arts, music, movement, and play activities. Rich and compelling descriptions of clinical work and research studies illustrate ways the creative arts, including drama, art, music, and movement therapies can support refugees as they process their experiences (Dieterich-Hartwell & Koch, 2017; Malchiodi, 2020). Expressive arts therapies can give culturally congruent ways of reconstructing meaning and coalescing new identities, while managing feelings of grief and loss for refugee children and families

The Home of Expressive Arts in Learning (HEAL) program reported positive outcomes for teen refugees through the use of art and music therapy (Quinlan et al., 2016). Play and time in nature can be facilitated by advocating for access to safe, child-friendly playgrounds, mobile play vehicles, parks, and green spaces.

## Play Therapy

Play therapy can be pivotal in creating a safe relational space and attuned pace to encounter traumatic memories from the migration process. Therapeutically guided play can help children and families shift from survivor to capable agent mode, improving feelings of self-efficacy, regulating arousal, and helping the child develop better coping strategies for fear-based, dysregulated responses (Prichard, 2016). Child-centered play therapy (CCPT) has been shown to provide refugee children with corrective experiences that counter traumatic experiences. Haas and Ray (2020) described positive outcomes at home and school for an 8-year-old refugee girl using CCPT. The intervention included consultations and psycho-educational meetings to share therapeutic skills with the child's mother and aunt, who served as cultural brokers.

## ATTACHMENT-BASED FAMILY THERAPY

Themes experienced by families during migration and resettlement include disrupted family norms, altered roles, and changed power structures (Bemak & Chung, 2021). Strengthening attachment bonds using family therapy and filial interventions are recommended approaches to help inoculate family relationships during the tumultuous post-migration adjustment process. The refugee experience can lead to intergenerational trauma, the transmission of emotional and neurobiological trauma responses between generations, primarily through the disruption of the attachment process between caregiver and child (Lim & Ogawa, 2014). Lim and Ogawa (2014) demonstrated that a relational shift between caregiver and child was possible through child–parent relationship therapy, leading to a reduction of both internalizing and externalizing symptoms for all family members.

## SCHOOL-BASED APPROACHES

In accordance with an ecological and systems-based approach, school-based interventions can provide effective support services to refugee children and their families. With the availability of on-site mental health support and interpreters, the school setting offers greater access to intervention. In addition, school personnel are frequently trained in the practice of cultural humility and trauma-informed care. Schools can cultivate partnerships with other community agencies, creating a more integrated network for services. When adjusting to post-migration transitions, children benefit from everyday life routines that are associated with resuming school.

Whether a provider is working with an individual or with the family, it is important to address psychosocial factors. These contextual dimensions gain prominence and influence successful progress during the post-migration phase.

## CASE EXAMPLES[3]

Refugees' journeys to resettlement vary widely and are fraught with danger and uncertainty at both personal and systemic levels. In this section, we will share scenarios depicting refugee experiences. After reading the scenarios, reflective prompts and questions are offered after the vignettes to support your exploration and integration of the information with your current knowledge, clinical skills, and practice of cultural humility. You are invited to use journaling and expressive arts, such as painting, collage-making, and movement, to support your journey. You are encouraged to find a partner or a small group to share your learning and reflections about the scenarios below:

---

[3] Case scenarios are based on current statistics regarding originating and host countries, causes of fleeing, and demographics of the refugees.

1. Dabir (25) and his partner Arif (23) fled their home in Syria due to threats of violence related to their identities and relationships. While living under the sustained threat of violence due to civil war, the couple faced hostility from their families and experienced daily discrimination within their community. They were forced to flee Syria when Arif's cousin threatened to kill Dabir. Though they escaped immediate danger in Syria, they experienced continued threats throughout their migration and upon reaching a neighboring country. Uncertain about when and where their resettlement placement will be, the couple hopes they will soon be able to live together in an accepting, affirming community.

2. Ajaa, along with her three children ages 9, 7, and 4, and her mother, Yusra, fled South Sudan due to escalating violence, food insecurity, and devastation to their village from flooding. Ajaa has not seen her husband since he was forced to fight in the war 2 years ago, and she fears that he has been killed. In an attempt to find safety, food, and shelter, Ajaa and Yusra decided to embark on a dangerous trek to a neighboring county. While journeying on foot, the family had limited water and food, and risked gender-based violence. As they await the processing of their application, Ajaa and Yusra struggle to access sufficient food and water and keep a watchful eye on the children in the camp due to the worries about unsafe sanitary conditions and child traffickers.

3. The Perez family had been diligently saving money so that all five members could leave their homes in Venezuela due to the poverty and economic hardship. Parents, Alejandra and Mauricio, were forced to make the challenging decision to separate their family when their 16-year-old son, Rafael, was put in significant danger due to escalating gang violence and the sudden lack of access to medication for his chronic medical condition. Leaving their two daughters in the care of Alejandra's sister, Rafael and his parents fled. They are eager to reunite their family and hope that upon resettling, they will be able to reunite with extended family members and reestablish their community of support.

## REFLECTIVE PROMPTS

For each scenario, consider the challenges faced by the persons at the time of arrival and anticipate the support needed to enhance the trajectory of their adjustment as you contemplate your role and possible intervention strategies.

- Imagine the persons arrived in your town. Would there be opportunities for them to meet other refugee, immigrant, and local families/couples? What do you know about how easy or difficult it would be for them to find work? How would the children be welcomed by their peers?

How challenging might it be for them to access adequate funding and guidance for housing, legal support, and other necessary relocation services from local and national organizations?

- What questions arise for you as you read about their situations during premigration and migration? How do you react to their envisioning of their lives post-migration? What do you want to know more about?
- Consider your cultural perspectives on health, wellness, and healing. How might they align with the client/family's perspectives? In what way might therapeutic intervention, including counseling, be viewed?
- Describe how you would determine what role you might play. You are encouraged to reflect on your identity, beliefs, and values. Would you defer being involved because of lack of knowledge or skills, consider referring to a different professional or agency? Might you serve in a consultative or coordination role, perhaps facilitating interprofessional team building with the resettlement liaison, medical and work/placement agencies, educational system, faith-based resources, or interpreters? Advocate at the systemic level to reduce barriers to treatment? Serve as a volunteer?
- If you determine you might serve as a direct service provider, what cultural humility-informed approaches and trauma-informed interventions come to mind? What supports will you benefit from?

As you move forward and consider possible ways to connect and support refugees, we encourage you to intentionally adopt a cultural humility-informed approach. This may mean that moving directly to "trauma work," as depicted in the professional literature, is contraindicated. Rather, reflect on your competencies, endeavor to prioritize your client's beliefs and identified concerns, look for systemic barriers to address, and engage with respect to build trusting relationships.

## FUTURE PROJECTIONS AND CONCERNS

Maintaining existing services and expanding efforts to support persons with refugee status are fraught with intersecting tides of political, environmental, economic, and regulatory uncertainty. Countries are facing high levels of food insecurity and malnutrition due to devastating record-high environmental events and conflicts within and between nations. Disparities in the media coverage and the response of the international community to refugees fleeing from humanitarian crises in different countries illuminate discriminatory biases in access to sustained support. Combined with widespread economic instability and the limited capacity of many countries to deliver basic services, the likelihood that the number of refugees will diminish soon is further reduced. Thus, there is a continued need for trained mental health providers to serve this population. Fortunately, many scholars and practitioners are developing culturally congruent interventions and frameworks to guide the efforts of mental health providers and organizations (Im et al., 2021).

## CONCLUSION

Refugees confront significant mental health challenges related to trauma, lack of access to culturally attuned medical and mental health services, disruption of their careers and education, social exclusion, and economic turmoil. Stressors can be expected to develop within a family as each person adapts at different speeds and with varying amounts of ease to the new cultural and linguistic norms and intervention efforts. Given the prevalence of psychological trauma for resettled refugees, it is crucial that we embody cultural humility and practice trauma-informed strategies, balancing effective clinical skills and traditional healing beliefs to enhance positive outcomes to meet the refugees' needs and support their family, work, and life trajectories. Clarissa Pinkola Estés (2020) offered a perspective we have found helpful in our work, "Ours is not the task of fixing the entire world at once, but of stretching out to mend the part of the world that is within our reach." Indeed.

## REFERENCES

Albers, T., Ariccio, S., Weiss, L. A., Dessi, F., & Bonaiuto, M. (2021). The role of place attachment in promoting refugees' well-being and resettlement: A literature review. *International Journal of Environmental Research and Public Health*, *18*(21), 11021. https://doi.org/10.3390/ijerph182111021

Bemak, F., & Chung, R. C.-Y. (2021). Contemporary refugees: Issues, challenges, and a culturally responsive intervention model for effective practice. *The Counseling Psychologist*, *49*(2), 305–324. https://doi.org/10.1177/0011000020972182

Carll, E., Chakaryan, H., & Stiles, D. (2021). *An overview of issues in working with vulnerable immigrant and refugee populations* [Webinar]. Refugee Mental Health Resource Network Webinar: An APA Interdivisional Project. https://www.apatraumadivision. org/527/webinar-series.html

Dieterich-Hartwell, R., & Koch, S. C. (2017). Creative arts therapies as temporary home for refugees: Insights from literature and practice. *Behavioral Science*, *7*(4), 69. https://doi.org/10.3390/bs7040069

Foverskov, E., White, J. S., Frøslev, T., Sørensen, H. T., & Hamad, R. (2022). Risk of psychiatric disorders among refugee children and adolescents living in disadvantaged neighborhoods. *JAMA Pediatrics*, *176*(11), 1107–1114. https://doi.org/ 10.1001/jamapediatrics.2022.3235

Frounfelker, R. L., Miconi, D., Farrar, J., Brooks, M. A., Rousseau, C., & Betancourt, T. S. (2020). Mental health of refugee children and youth: Epidemiology, interventions, and future directions. *Annual Review of Public Health*, *41*, 159–176. https://doi.org/ 10.1146/annurev-publhealth-040119-094230

Gwozdziewycs, N., & Mehl-Madrona, L. (2013). Meta-analysis of the use of narrative exposure therapy for the effects of trauma among refugee populations. *The Permanente Journal, 17*(1), 72–78. https://doi.org/10.7812/TPP/12-058

Haas, S. C., & Ray, D. C. (2020). Child-centered play therapy with children affected by adverse childhood experiences: A single-case design. *International Journal of Play Therapy, 29*(4), 223–236. https://doi.org/10.1037/pla0000135

Hilado, A., Reznicek, E., & Allweiss, S. (2021). Primer on understanding the refugee experience. In J. D. Aten & J. Hwang (Eds.), *Refugee mental health* (pp. 19–43). American Psychological Association. https://doi.org/10.1037/0000226-002

Im, H., Rodriguez, C., & Grumbine, J. M. (2021). A multitier model of refugee mental health and psychosocial support in resettlement: Toward trauma-informed and culture-informed systems of care. *Psychological Services, 18*(3), 345–364. https://doi.org/10.1037/ser0000412

Lely, J. C., Smid, G. E., Jongedijk, R. A., Knipscheer, J. W., & Kleber, R. J. (2019). The effectiveness of narrative exposure therapy: a review, meta-analysis and meta-regression analysis. *European Journal of Psychotraumatology, 10*(1), 1550344. https://doi.org/10.1080/20008198.2018.1550344

Lim, S.-L., & Ogawa, Y. (2014). "Once I had kids, now I am raising kids": Child-Parent Relationship Therapy (CPRT) with a Sudanese refugee family—A case study. *International Journal of Play Therapy, 23*(2), 70–89. https://doi.org/10.1037/a0036362

Malchiodi, C. (2020). *Trauma and expressive arts therapy: Brain, body, and imagination in the healing process.* The Guilford Press.

Murray-Garcia, J., & Tervalon, M. (2017). Rethinking intercultural competence: Cultural humility in internationalising higher education. In D. Deardorff & L. Arasaratnam-Smith (Eds.), *Intercultural competence in higher education: International approaches, assessments, and application.* Routledge.

Nosè, M., Ballette, F., Bighelli, I., Turrini, G., Purgato, M., Tol, W., Priebe, S., & Barbui, C. (2017). Psychosocial interventions for post-traumatic stress disorder in refugees and asylum seekers resettled in high-income countries: Systematic review and meta-analysis. *PLoS One, 12*(2). https://doi.org/10.1371/journal.pone.0171030

O'Brien, C. V., & Charura, D. (2022). Refugees, asylum seekers, and practitioners' perspectives of embodied trauma: A comprehensive scoping review. *Psychological Trauma Theory Research Practice and Policy.* https://doi.org/10.1037/tra0001342

Perry, B. D. (2006). Applying principles of neurodevelopment to clinical work with maltreated and traumatized children: The neurosequential model of therapeutics. In N. B. Webb (Ed.), *Working with traumatized youth in child welfare* (pp. 27–52). The Guilford Press.

Pinkola Estés, C. (2020). *Do not lose heart, we were made for these times.* Denver Westword. https://www.westword.com/news/clarissa-pinkola-estes-do-not-lose-heart-we-were-made-for-these-times-11677029

Porges, S. W. (2011). *The polyvagal theory: Neurophysiological foundations of emotions, attachment, communication, and self-regulation.* W.W. Norton & Company.

Prichard, N. (2016). Stuck in the dollhouse: A brain-based perspective of post-traumatic play. In D. Le Vay & E. Cuschieri (Eds.), *Challenges in the theory and practice of play therapy* (pp. 71–85). Routledge/Taylor & Francis Group.

Quinlan, R., Schweitzer, R. D., Khawaja, N., & Griffin, J. (2016). Evaluation of a school-based creative arts therapy program for adolescents from refugee backgrounds. *The Arts in Psychotherapy, 47,* 72–78.

Substance Abuse and Mental Health Services Administration. (2014). *Trauma-informed care in behavioral health services: Treatment improvement protocol (TIP) series 57* (SMA 14-4816). https://www.ncbi.nlm.nih.gov/books/NBK207201/pdf/Bookshelf_NBK207201.pdf

Umer, M., & Elliot, D. L. (2018). Being hopeful: Exploring the dynamics of post-traumatic growth and hope in refugees. *Journal of Refugee Studies, 34*(1), 953–975. https://doi.org/10.1093/jrs/fez002

United Nations High Commissioner for Refugees. (2023). *USA for UNHCR: The UN refugee agency.* https://www.unrefugees.org/

United Nations International Organization for Migration. (2023). *IOM UN migration: About migration.* https://www.iom.int/about-migration

Unterhitzenberger, J., Eberle-Sejari, R., Rassenhofer, M., Sukale, T., Rosner, R., & Goldbeck, L. (2015). Trauma-focused cognitive behavioral therapy with unaccompanied refugee minors: A case series. *BMC Psychiatry, 15,* 260. https://doi.org/10.1186/s12888-015-0645-0

Vindevogel, S., & Verelst, A. (2020). Supporting mental health in young refugees: A resilience perspective. In S. J. Song & P. Ventevogel (Eds.), *Child, adolescent and family refugee mental: A global perspective* (pp. 53–65). Springer. https://doi.org/10.1007/978-3-030-45278-0_4

## CHAPTER TWELVE

# Impacts of Attachment Trauma on Children in Foster or Adoptive Care

PARIS GOODYEAR-BROWN and THERESA FRASER

## INTRODUCTION

This chapter explores attachment traumas occurring in foster and adoptive populations. The process of adoption involves a series of initial traumatic experiences for the child, including potential in utero developmental injuries, abrupt caregiver disruptions, a felt sense of betrayal, abandonment, or rejection, and often, time spent in institutions where there are limited serve-and-return experiences. These initial attachment ruptures set the stage for a host of secondary trauma dynamics in adoptive children. Secondary trauma, defined as a subsequent breakdown in the survivors' sense of self in relationship to others, (Catsherall, 1989) may include impaired attachment capacities, extreme difficulty in trusting others, long-term difficulties in social relationships, and neurophysiological dysregulation that can negatively impact the feedback that the child receives within a multitude of developmental areas. This chapter provides a case example and identifies effective treatments for both initial trauma targets and secondary trauma targets.

*Trauma Impacts: The Repercussions of Individual and Collective Trauma*, First Edition.
Edited by Jessica Stone, Robert J. Grant, and Clair Mellenthin.

## IN UTERO THREATS: EXCESS CORTISOL TIED TO INTERPERSONAL VIOLENCE, DRUGS, AND ALCOHOL

The developing child's story begins in utero, as the umbilical cord becomes the conduit for fetal programming (Kwon & Kim, 2017). Oxygen, nutrients, stress hormones (maternal endogenous cortisol), and other threats such as drugs and alcohol can travel in the mother's blood via the umbilical cord to the developing fetus. Waste products, including carbon monoxide, travel back to the mother's circulation via the placenta and umbilical cord (Heil & Bordoni, 2022). Pathways for the transmission of stress hormones through gene–environment interactions, epigenetics, and specific mechanisms, such as the hypothalamic–pituitary–adrenal axis and cytokines, are adding weight to the powerful role of in utero experiences in creating a traumatic or welcoming beginning to the human experience (Glover et al., 2018; Verny & Kelly, 1982).

Normative levels of cortisol help a baby to grow; however, cortisol can become neurotoxic to the baby's brain development in excess amounts (Nath et al., 2017). When a birth mother makes the decision to place her baby up for adoption, it is likely that she has experienced greater than normal amounts of stress, and therefore cortisol production, during key moments of the baby's development. This stress may stem from a lack of resources (emotional, financial, family, or societal support), a lack of emotional readiness, the stress involved with hiding a pregnancy, ongoing experiences of interpersonal violence, substance use, or other traumatic life circumstances. Once the mother has made the decision to terminate parental rights, she may also experience the stressful effects of grief, loss, guilt, shame, and so on.

The experience of intimate partner violence (IPV) generates subsequent higher than normal levels of cortisol within the mother's bloodstream and is associated with low infant weight gain. Chronic maternal stress leads to increased fetal cortisol, glucose, and insulin resistance (Valsamakis et al., 2020). IPV can also negatively impact the mother's ability to regularly attend prenatal, perinatal, or personal medical appointments (Alhusen et al., 2015).

Violence or the threat of violence toward the mother is followed by excessive cortisol production, which can damage the developing regulation structures of the autonomic nervous system (ANS) within the fetus, while also triggering mental health issues in the mother. Perinatal mothers who are also IPV survivors are at an increased risk of mother-to-infant bonding failure and the use of faulty coping strategies, such as substance use (Mazza et al., 2021), all of which can lead to impairments in the neurophysiological regulation of the developing child.

A woman may be exposed to alcohol during periods of critical embryologic development before she even knows that she is pregnant. The brain can be impacted at any stage of pregnancy and even during breastfeeding when neurogenesis of brain cells is occurring, which can thus lead to future cognitive and behavioral challenges. The most recent version of the Diagnostic and Statistical Manual (American Psychiatric Association, 2022) introduced the diagnosis Neurobehavioral Disorder Associated with Prenatal Alcohol Exposure (ND-PAE) meant to capture the multitude of developmental differences that can result from alcohol use in utero. The symptoms include impaired neurocognitive functioning, self-regulation deficits (i.e., attention deficits, mood disorders, and poor impulse control), and impairment in adaptive functioning (i.e., impaired language skills and social skills deficits). Fetal Alcohol Spectrum Disorder (FASD) is marked by growth deficits, birth defects, and neurodevelopmental impairments (Kaminen-Ahola, 2020; Tan et al., 2015). Recent epidemics of opioid and methamphetamine addictions have resulted in a generation of babies who have damaged neurological regulation systems and have become addicted in utero. When an infant is removed from a mother's care at the hospital due to substance use issues, infants suffer injury upon injury: the loss of their attachment figure at the very time that they are also experiencing painful withdrawals from the substances upon which they became dependent during pregnancy.

## ABRUPT CAREGIVER DISRUPTIONS
## AND BETRAYAL TRAUMA

Near-term babies and newborns recognize and discriminate between their mother's voice and the voice of others (Abrams et al., 2016; DeCasper & Fifer, 1980; Voegtline et al., 2013). It is believed that babies also recognize the smell of their mother. Their olfactory receptor neurons begin to develop at week 6 gestationally, and magnetic resonance imaging testing shows that by 30 weeks, the growing baby can distinguish between smells (Sarnat et al., 2017). In recent studies, infants have evidenced recognition of their own mother's breast milk through a decrease in pain indicators (heart rate, oxygen saturation, and blood pressure) (Rad et al., 2021) and movement toward their mother's breast odor (crawling and head rooting) (Hym et al., 2021; Tristão et al., 2021).

Infants can recognize their biological parents. Infants can also recognize when they are separated from their parents. When a newborn is confronted with unfamiliar smells and unfamiliar voices during the hours and days after birth, the work of adjusting to the world outside of the womb is much harder. Abrupt abandonment is experienced on the sensory self by the infant.

The newborn's neurophysiology is primed for immediate soothing by the mother, and this sudden loss of familiar sounds and smells can lead to a series of implicit memories of loss and dysregulation, fueling a neuroception of danger instead of safety.

Children who are separated from their primary attachment figure may experience an initial betrayal trauma (mainly encoded in implicit memory systems), and revisit and re-story this trauma as they move through different developmental stages. Freyd (1996) defines *betrayal trauma* as a trauma that occurs after an individual is violated because the institution or individuals that were identified to meet their needs do not do so. Whether a child is removed from their parent's care due to neglect or abuse or intentionally placed with a foster or adoption agency, the child experiences a core betrayal of being left by the person who was meant to be their caregiver. The attachment disruption itself is a primary trauma accompanied by sequela injuries, such as grief and loss, potential abuse or neglect in subsequent placements, and the lack of attuned caregiving. These experiences impede the child's development of a fundamental sense of self as good and worthy of love and connection. A secondary trauma dynamic ensues in which a child is continually questioning their core identity, their core right to exist, their innate human right to give and receive love, and to belong.

Disruption in the initial caregiving relationship happens in all cultures and at all socioeconomic levels; however, from a macrosystemic perspective, marginalized people groups experience greater caregiver disruptions than the general public. Institutional oppression leads to difficulty accessing higher education, which leads to difficulty in securing high-paying jobs. The dynamics of poverty lead to parents who are working long hours, sometimes working two or more jobs while having limited access to childcare. Disenfranchised parents lack access to multiple resources, including access to high-quality health care and quality counseling services, and may have easy access to illicit drugs while having little access to substance abuse programs that work. Parents who live in poverty are faced with the daily toxic stressors of racism, sexism, and classism, while living in neighborhoods that are riddled with crime. This begs the question: How do we create systemic changes that support all families? Victims of betrayal trauma may also be fearful of disclosing their experiences for fear that future needs and even attachment relationships are at risk (Reyes et al., 2008). Adoption is only possible in the wake of the loss of a primary attachment figure. While this fundamental attachment trauma engenders the adoptee's return to questions of self-worth and trust at various stages of development, adoptive children can feel pressured to seem grateful for their rescue, and adoptive parents can unintentionally minimize the pain of the child's grief over the lost parent(s).

## EFFECTS OF INSTITUTIONAL CARE

An institutional care setting will not likely provide children with the quantity and dosing of attuned interactions with a primary caregiver that a single-family unit can provide. In these settings, both attention and resources must be shared among multiple children and few caregivers. This ratio can be as large as 10 children to 1 caregiver (Hecker et al., 2021). In the first six months of life, infants are the most vulnerable to the effects of institutionalization (Bronfenbrenner, 1979), which can include diminished "physical resources, unfavorable and unstable staffing patterns, and social-emotionally inadequate caregiver-child interactions" (van IJzendoorn et al., 2011, p. 8). Developmentally supportive environments, such as family placements, are less likely to perpetuate the effects of institutionalized settings (Julian, 2013). Social, emotional, physical, and cognitive functioning can improve in such settings and Reactive Attachment Disorder (RAD) can be mitigated (Guyon-Harris et al., 2019). However, children could still be at risk to demonstrate ongoing behavioral challenges (Pollak et al., 2010), particularly if they experience betrayal trauma.

## ATTACHMENT IMPAIRMENTS

Children come into the world hardwired for connection with their caregivers. Attachment depends on the infant experiencing caregivers' responses to meeting their needs (Bowlby, 1958). If the child does not experience the activation of their attachment system, it is believed that future attachment formation is at risk (Sullivan, 2012). Lifelong attachment capacities are being wired into the neurophysiology of newborns and the serve-and-return communication between mothers and their babies becomes the dance of co-regulation, with co-regulation by a caregiver always precedes self-regulation (Goodyear-Brown, 2021, 2022).

Traumatized mothers are at risk for developing a variety of mood and anxiety disorders during the perinatal period (Beydoun et al., 2010; Muzik et al., 2016; Oh et al., 2016). Depression, post-traumatic stress disorder (PTSD), and the trauma associated with IPV all compromise the mother's availability to sensitively and contingently respond to her baby (Schechter et al., 2005). Blunted affect, a lack of prosodic variability in the mother's voice, withdrawn, dissociated, or slowed responses, or negative activation can lead to a lack of attuned responsiveness between mothers and their newborns and may lead to mother-to-infant bonding failure.

Feeney (2005) states, "Adoption may be a risk factor for later attachment insecurity and suggests that it is worth examining the impact of insecurity on the adoptee's relational attitudes and behaviors" (p. 46). Loss, rejection, shame, guilt, grief, identity, intimacy, mastery, and control are considered the seven core issues of adoption (Roszia & Maxon, 2019). These set the stage for secondary trauma dynamics, including a breakdown in survivors' sense of self (Catsherall, 1989), and may include impaired attachment capacities, extreme difficulty trusting others, long-term difficulties in social relationships, and neurophysiological dysregulation that can negatively impact the feedback that the child receives in a multitude of developmental areas.

## IMPLICATIONS FOR ADOPTIVE FAMILIES

Children who have experienced attachment disruptions can struggle with parent and sibling relationships. Foster and adoptive parents report that their children do not trust that the parents will meet their needs. These children are unlikely to ask for concrete or emotional resources. In fact, children with attachment disruptions may go out of their way to solve their own challenges and avoid being viewed as having an unmet need even when it is developmentally appropriate to have such a need. They may hoard food, lie, cheat, and steal to ensure that they are not dependent on caregivers. Many children with insecure attachments develop the core belief *I must control everything at all costs because I cannot trust anyone else to meet my needs*. The core belief of some is more profoundly stated as *I must control everything at all costs, or I will die*. These children develop a control foundation instead of a trust foundation. Admitting a dependence on an adult can trigger feelings of terror, shame, and weakness in the child. Corrective emotional experiences must be carefully approached, often therapeutically, by repeatedly pairing resources with the relationship (Goodyear-Brown, 2021).

Children who have lacked nurturing touch may have an aversion to even a light touch and may perceive physical touch to be controlling or painful. Caregivers can perceive their child's discomfort with touch as rejection and respond with withdrawal or force, which can create additional ruptures in building trust. Children may also lack an understanding of social boundaries. They may interact with strangers or external family members in overly familiar ways and may even put themselves at risk. Due to the inherent secrecy around sexual abuse, there are no clear statistics on the rates of sexual abuse in institutional settings, but children who have spent time in orphanages may have poor boundaries around touch and may need practice with setting and keeping safe touch boundaries within their adoptive homes.

Sexually reactive behaviors between a foster or adoptive child and other children in the home are a leading cause of adoption disruptions, with the abrupt removal causing yet another attachment trauma. It is critical that foster and adoptive caregivers be trained in how to supervise children with such vulnerabilities and how to address them through a trauma-informed lens. These children may also neglect to communicate responsibility for their actions and may not experience embarrassment or feel the need to engage in restorative interactions.

Without support and intervention, caregivers can report parenting experiences that leave them feeling incapable of bonding with their children. Siblings of adopted or foster children can report that they feel ignored, unsupported, or angry. They may even feel unworthy of adult attention because they recognize that their chosen siblings have a complexity of traumagenic experiences with which they can never compete. In some cases, the foster or adoptive child will destroy a biological child's possessions and physically hurt or bully other children in the home.

## TREATMENT NEEDS

Treatment needs of foster and adoptive families may include enhancing safety and security, assessing for and augmenting adaptive coping, helping caregivers shift their parenting paradigms for these children, building trust between children and caregivers, facilitating in vivo delighting-in experiences, expanding co-regulation and self-regulation skills, helping children ask for what they need, building coherent narratives around their birth parents, their culture, the story of their adoption, stories of belonging and stories around traumatic events, and stories that help to shift core beliefs about self and others toward health (Lind et al., 2019). TraumaPlay™, a flexibly sequential, components-based play therapy model for traumatized children and their families, which integrates several important therapeutic goals for working with this population (Goodyear-Brown, 2009, 2019) and will be demonstrated in the case example. The heart of TraumaPlay is to *follow the child's needs* throughout a continuum of treatment, integrating many different evidence-based approaches to further a developmental healing process that moves from regulation to connection to reason. The therapist functions in three rotating roles throughout treatment: Safe Boss, Nurturer, and Storykeeper, and helps parents to further embody these roles for the traumatized children in their care.

## CASE EXAMPLE

Leslie had two biological parents with developmental delays and had experienced nine moves before the age of seven. She experienced three foster placements, three returns to her parent's home, and two adoptive placement disruptions. Court affidavits indicated that Leslie experienced neglect and physical abuse. She was also encouraged by her father to lock her younger siblings in a dark basement and hit them when they would not stop crying. If she did not comply with her father's demands (per her later report), she herself would be locked in the basement alone with a scary doll.

After being expelled from kindergarten for sexually acting out on other children in her school bathroom, she was placed in a new foster family. She became the youngest of six children in the home. Leslie's third foster father was a stay-at-home dad, and after six weeks of one-on-one time with him (and an activity-filled summer with her foster siblings), she was placed in a first-grade classroom. Leslie was often sent home, at least twice a week, in response to the following big behaviors: defiance, disrespect, destruction of school property, and blurting out racist comments to teachers and peers alike.

Leslie slept little and argued regularly with her foster siblings. She was also aggressive with the family dog. Foster parents advocated for assessment, and she was subsequently diagnosed with RAD. The diagnosis precipitated her placement in a specialized classroom. However, even with two-to-one staffing and a classroom of only three peers, Leslie continued to be sent home at least twice a week when she was in second grade. She spent long periods of time in a padded, calm-down room by herself. The foster parents decided to move to a different state/province at the same time they decided to adopt her. Leslie was resistant to this idea due to her two previously failed adoptions. Therapy began after their move and consisted of once-weekly neurofeedback sessions coupled with Child-Centered Play Therapy (CCPT). CCPT is an effective way to meet the TraumaPlay™ goal of enhancing safety and security. When Leslie engaged in CCPT, she was first drawn to the babies and the food area of the playroom. She would make food for the therapist and care for the babies. Later, as a filial approach invited her mother or father to join the sessions, and she recapitulated these themes with her parents.

Concurrently, the therapist had collateral sessions with the parents, equipping them to become partners in the healing process. Parents were provided with psychoeducation about the impact of traumatic experiences on attachment and development, as well as co-regulation strategies and techniques for enhancing their own and the client's adaptive coping skills (Goodyear-Brown, 2009, 2019). It was necessary to prepare them for the ups and downs of trauma therapy. It was hypothesized that the closer Leslie got to her trauma memories, she would likely show her discomfort behaviorally. Parents were taught co-regulation skills, expanded their reflective capacity, and were prepared to help in the process of coherent narrative building.

The neurofeedback appeared to positively impact Leslie's sleep cycle. Adoptive parents also reported less examples of dysregulation, though there were continued episodes of property damage and food hoarding. Once safety was established and coping enhanced, the focus shifted to the TraumaPlay goal of soothing the physiology. Leslie also engaged in sensory motor arousal activities that would engage her vestibular, proprioceptive, and tactile sensory systems.

When she had sessions alone with the therapist, she was often drawn to the sand tray where she initially created scenes of conflict until these became scenes of discovery, where sand tray animals were searching for basic needs as a group in wild and dangerous lands. These worlds seem to reflect her openness to sharing her basic needs with family members. This was a new experience for her parents, who viewed her requests as evidence of attachment beginning between them. As therapy progressed, Leslie began to share stories of her past, mostly involving experiences with caregivers that reinforced her core belief that she had to do things all by herself. She would utilize the dollhouse on these occasions while showing the therapist what being locked in a basement might feel like. Handcuffs were also utilized on occasion. Leslie could eventually verbalize that she wished that she became part of her current family earlier in her life because they taught her that none of her past rejections were her fault, but rather coping behaviors to protect her from additional hurt. She began inviting her parents to hear the sand tray stories, illustrating her desire for them to become Storykeepers of her life narrative.

Eventually, she eagerly desired to have her parents in session with her. The therapist, following the child's need, pivoted to Theraplay(c) and began offering delighting-in games during sessions, working specifically on the domains of engagement and structure. Leslie had participated in Theraplay(c) with a previous foster parent, and the onset of a new round of work triggered some big behaviors at home. Dad was able to verbalize that he was feeling reactive to her tantrums, was having trouble sleeping, and wanting to avoid interaction and contact. The therapist invited dad to engage in three levels of the Safe and Sound Protocol for a total of 15 hours. Upon completion, Dad endorsed feeling less reactive to Leslie's attempts to target him. When Theraplay(c) ended, Leslie and her new parents were ready to say goodbye. Check-up and booster sessions were offered, as well as parent consultation as needed.

## SYSTEMIC ISSUES AND FUTURE RAMIFICATIONS

During the COVID-19 pandemic, between 2019 and 2020, the National Adoption Council (2021) reported a decrease in adoption rates in the United States. Private domestic, non-stepparent adoptions declined by 24%, intercountry adoptions declined by 45%, and adoptions from foster care declined by 13%. During this same time frame, unprecedented numbers of parents died from COVID-19 infections, leaving an unparalleled global orphan crisis. Adoption agencies and governmental organizations need to streamline the process of pairing parents and children together in forever homes. The longer an infant or toddler languishes in an institution or is moved around between multiple foster placements, the more likely the child is to experience neurophysiological dysregulation. Subsequently, the child and their caregivers are likely to need more medical, behavioral, psychological, and pharmacological help. This pattern further taxes the institutional care systems themselves, the child welfare system at large, and the global mental health care infrastructure. Children in foster and adoptive care who do not get the services that they need often end up in the criminal justice system, adding to the massive overload of these systems. Macrosystemic influences must prioritize the need for vulnerable children to be paired with Safe Bosses quickly and effectively. Exosystems can work to become more trauma-informed, offering enriching environments and intentional doses of serve-and-return communications with primary caregivers. Microsystems must work to equip foster and adoptive parents, both pre-placement and ongoing, with effective support to shift their paradigms toward trauma-informed parenting practices, while creating access to connected communities of parents facing similar situations.

## CONCLUSION

Institutional oppression, poverty, and limited access to resources set birth parents up to be at an increased risk for depression, anxiety, IPV, and drug and alcohol use. These challenges can result in children being separated from their birth parents. Attachment trauma that includes the loss of the first parent and placement in foster or adoptive care results in vulnerable children at risk for a lifetime of troubled relationships. Therapists and other professionals working with this population need to be cognizant that resources provided early can prevent more costly and intensive resources later. Targeted interventions and consistent communities of care can bring change at every level in order to better serve the next generation of foster and adoptive children and their caregivers.

## REFERENCES

Abrams, D. A., Chen, T., Odriozola, P., & Menon, V. (2016). Neural circuits underlying mother's voice perception predict social communication abilities in children. *PNAS, 113*(22), 6295–6300. https://doi.org/10.1073/pnas.160294811

Alhusen, J. L., Ray, E., Sharps, P., & Bullock, L. (2015). Intimate partner violence during pregnancy: Maternal and neonatal outcomes. *Journal of Women's Health, 24*(1), 100–106. https://doi.org/10.1089/jwh.2014.4872

American Psychiatric Association (2022). *Diagnostic and statistical manual of mental disorders* (5th ed.). https://doi.org/10.1176/appi.books.9780890425596

Beydoun, H. A., Al-Sahab, B., Beydoun, M. A., & Tamim, H. (2010). Intimate partner violence as a risk factor for postpartum depression among Canadian women in the maternity experience survey. *Annals of Epidemiology, 20*(8), 575–583.

Bowlby, J. (1958). The nature of the child's tie to his mother. In P. M. D. Buckley (Red.), *Essential papers on object relations* (pp. 350—373). New York University Press.

Bronfenbrenner, U. (1979). *The ecology of human development: Experiments by nature and design.* Harvard University Press.

Catsherall, D. R. (1989). Differentiating intervention strategies for primary and secondary trauma in post-traumatic stress disorder: The example of Vietnam veterans. *Journal of Traumatic Stress, 2*(3), 289–304.

DeCasper, A. J., & Fifer, W. P. (1980). Of human bonding: Newborns prefer their mothers' voices. *Science, 208*(4448), 1174–1176.

Feeney, J. (2005). Attachment and perceived rejection: Findings from studies of hurt feelings and the adoption experience. *E-Journal of Applied Psychology, 1*(1), 41–49.

Freyd, J. J. (1996). *Betrayal trauma: The logic of forgetting childhood abuse.* Harvard University Press.

Glover, V., O'Donnell, K., O'Connor, T., & Fisher, J. (2018). Prenatal maternal stress, fetal programming, and mechanisms underlying later psychopathology—A global perspective. *Development and Psychopathology, 30*(3), 843–854.

Goodyear-Brown, P. (2009). *Play therapy with traumatized children: A prescriptive approach.* John Wiley and Sons.

Goodyear-Brown, P. (2019). *Trauma and play therapy: Helping children heal.* Routledge.

Goodyear-Brown, P. (2021). *Parents as partners in child therapy: A clinician's guide.* Guilford Press.

Goodyear-Brown, P. (2022). *Big behaviors in small containers.* PESI.

Guyon-Harris, K. L., Humphreys, K. L., Degnan, K., Fox, N. A., Nelson, C. A., & Zeanah, C. H. (2019). A prospective longitudinal study of reactive attachment disorder following early institutional care: Considering variable-and person-centered approaches. *Attachment & Human Development, 21*(2), 95–110.

Hecker, T., Mkinga, G., Kirika, A., Nkuba, M., Preston, J., & Hermenau, K. (2021). Preventing maltreatment in institutional care: A cluster-randomized controlled trial in East Africa. *Preventive Medicine Reports, 24*, 101593.

Heil, J. R., & Bordoni, B. (2022). *Embryology, umbilical cord.* StatPearls Publishing.

Hym, C., Forma, V., Anderson, D. I., Provasi, J., Granjon, L., Huet, V., Carpe, E., Teulier, C., Durand, K., Schaal, B., & Barbu-Roth, M. (2021). Newborn crawling and rooting in response to maternal breast odor. *Developmental Science, 24*(3), e13061.

van IJzendoorn, M. H., Palacios, J., Sonuga-Barke, E. J., Gunnar, M. R., Vorria, P., McCall, R. B., LeMare, L., Bakermans-Kranenburg, M. J., Dobrova-Krol, N. A., & Juffer, F. (2011). Children in institutional care: Delayed development and resilience. *Monographs of the Society for Research in Child Development, 76*(4), 8–30.

Julian, M. M. (2013). Age at adoption from institutional care as a window into the lasting effects of early experiences. *Clinical Child and Family Psychology Review, 16*(2), 101–145.

Kaminen-Ahola, N. (2020). Fetal alcohol spectrum disorders: Genetic and epigenetic mechanisms. *Prenatal Diagnosis, 40*(9), 1185–1192.

Kwon, E. J., & Kim, Y. J. (2017). What is fetal programming?: A lifetime health is under the control of in utero health. *Obstetrics & Gynecology Science, 60*(6), 506–519.

Lind, M., Vanwoerden, S., Penner, F., & Sharp, C. (2019). Inpatient adolescents with borderline personality disorder features: Identity diffusion and narrative incoherence. *Personality Disorders, Theory, Research, and Treatment, 10*(4), 389–393. https://doi.org/10.1037/per0000338

Mazza, M., Caroppo, E., Marano, G., Chieffo, D., Moccia, L., Janiri, D., Rinaldi, L., Janiri, L., & Sani, G. (2021). Caring for mothers: A narrative review on interpersonal violence and peripartum mental health. *International Journal of Environmental Research and Public Health, 18*(10), 5281.

Muzik, M., McGinnis, E. W., Bocknek, E., Morelen, D., Rosenblum, K. L., Liberzon, I., Seng, J., & Abelson, J. L. (2016). PTSD symptoms across pregnancy and early postpartum among women with lifetime PTSD diagnosis. *Depression and Anxiety, 33*(7), 584–591.

Nath, A., Murthy, G. V. S., Babu, G. R., & Di Renzo, G. C. (2017). Effect of prenatal exposure to maternal cortisol and psychological distress on infant development in Bengaluru, southern India: A prospective cohort study. *BMC Psychiatry, 17*(1), 1–6.

National Council for Adoption. (2021, February 8). *ThemeNcode PDF Viewer SC—National Council For Adoption.* https://adoptioncouncil.org/themencode-pdf-viewer-sc/?tnc_pvfw=ZmlsZT1odHRwczovL2Fkb3B0aW9uY291bmNpbC5vcmcvY29udGVudC91cGxvYWRzLzIwMjIvMTIvQWRvcHRpb24tYnktdGhlLU51bWJlcnMtTmF0aW9uYWwtQ291bmNpbC1Gb3ItQWRvcHRpb24tRGVjLTIwMjIucGRmJnNldHRpbmdzPTExMTAxMDExMA

Oh, W., Muzik, M., McGinnis, E. W., Hamilton, L., Menke, R. A., & Rosenblum, K. L. (2016). Comorbid trajectories of postpartum depression and PTSD among mothers with childhood trauma history: Course, predictors, processes and child adjustment. *Journal of Affective Disorders, 200*, 133–141.

Pollak, S. D., Nelson, C. A., Schlaak, M. F., Roeber, B. J., Wewerka, S. S., Wiik, K. L., Frenn, K. A., Loman, M. M., & Gunnar, M. R. (2010). Neurodevelopmental effects of early deprivation in post institutionalized children. *Child Development, 81*(1), 224–236.

Rad, Z. A., Aziznejadroshan, P., Amiri, A. S., Ahangar, H. G., & Valizadehchari, Z. (2021). The effect of inhaling mother's breast milk odor on the behavioral responses to pain caused by hepatitis B vaccine in preterm infants: A randomized clinical trial. *BMC Pediatrics, 21*(1), 1–6.

Reyes, G., Elhai, J. D., & Ford, J. D. (Eds.) (2008). *The encyclopedia of psychological trauma.* Wiley.

Roszia, S., & Maxon, A. D. (2019). *Seven core issues in adoption and permanency: A comprehensive guide to promoting understanding and healing in adoption, foster care, kinship families and third party reproduction.* Jessica Kingsley Publishers.

Sarnat, H. B., Flores-Sarnat, L., & Wei, X. C. (2017). Olfactory development, part 1: Function, from fetal perception to adult wine-tasting. *Journal of Child Neurology, 32*(6), 566–578.

Schechter, D. S., Coots, T., Zeanah, C. H., Davies, M. G., Coates, S. W., Trabka, K. A., Marshall, R. D., Liebowitz, M. R., & Myers, M. D. (2005). Maternal mental representations of the child in an inner-city clinical sample: Violence-related posttraumatic stress and reflective functioning. *Attachment & Human Development, 7*(3), 313–331. https://doi.org/10.1080/14616730500246011

Sullivan, R. M. (2012). The neurobiology of attachment to nurturing and abusive caregivers. *The Hastings Law Journal, 63*(6), 1553–1570.

Tan, C. H., Denny, C. H., Cheal, N. E., Sniezek, J. E., & Kanny, D. (2015). Alcohol use and binge drinking among women of childbearing age—United States, 2011–2013. *Morbidity and Mortality Weekly Report, 64*(37), 1042–1046.

Tristão, R. M., Lauand, L., Costa, K. S. F., Brant, L. A., Fernandes, G. M., Costa, K. N., Brant, L. A., Fernandes, G. M., Costa, K. N., Spilski, J., & Lachmann, T. (2021). Olfactory sensory and perceptual evaluation in newborn infants: A systematic review. *Developmental Psychobiology, 63*(7), e22201.

Valsamakis, G., Papatheodorou, D., Chalarakis, N., Manolikaki, M., Margeli, A., Papassotiriou, I., Barber, T. M., Kumar, S., Kalantaridou, S., & Mastorakos, G. (2020). Maternal chronic stress correlates with serum levels of cortisol, glucose and C-peptide in the fetus, and maternal non chronic stress with fetal growth. *Psychoneuroendocrinology, 114*, e104591.

Verny, T., & Kelly, J. (1982). *The secret life of the unborn child: How you can prepare your baby for a happy, healthy life.* Dell.

Voegtline, K. M., Costigan, K. A., Pater, H. A., & DiPietro, J. A. (2013). Near-term fetal response to maternal spoken voice. *Infant Behavior & Development, 36*(4), 526–533.

## CHAPTER THIRTEEN

# When the Helper is in Crisis, Too

LISA DION

## THE HELPER

People working in "helping professions" are called to the front line to offer support on all levels: individual, community, national, and even international crises. These "helpers" consist of first responders, therapists, social workers, healthcare professionals, teachers, clergy, and any other individual who offers support during or after a traumatic event (Stamm et al., 2002). Helpers are a unique group of individuals, as they choose professions that directly put themselves to situations of trauma exposure. They are asked to listen, witness, and in many cases, experience the trauma alongside those they are helping. This places helpers in a position of great importance for those who need them while simultaneously increasing their own vulnerability to the effects of trauma.

In addition to trauma exposure by way of helping others, helpers also have their own history of traumatic experiences. According to national scientific studies, about 50% of women and 60% of men in the United States are exposed to potentially traumatizing events in their life (Stamm et al., 2002). The Adverse Childhood Experiences (ACEs) studies found that 61% of adults had at least one ACE and 16% had four or more types of ACEs (Center for Disease Control, 2021). Since the COVID-19 pandemic, these statistics have likely increased. This means that the probability of the helper also having had their own traumatic experiences is high. Another important consideration unique

*Trauma Impacts: The Repercussions of Individual and Collective Trauma*, First Edition.
Edited by Jessica Stone, Robert J. Grant, and Clair Mellenthin.
© 2024 John Wiley & Sons, Inc. Published 2024 by John Wiley & Sons, Inc.

to the field of crisis work is that many helpers feel driven to dedicate their careers to helping others due to their own history of trauma exposure and experiences.

This chapter aims to address the impact of trauma on the helper by looking at the following critical questions: What happens when the helper has experienced first or secondary trauma? How do the traumatic experiences of the impacted helper affect their ability to help and what is the potential impact on the person they are trying to help? How does a helper navigate their own unresolved trauma when it is activated while helping? Finally, this chapter will explore what can be done to mitigate the impact of trauma exposure, including new ideas from Interpersonal Neurobiology (Siegel, 2020) and Polyvagal Theory (Porges, 2021), allowing the helper to continue to thrive in this incredibly important role.

## PSYCHOLOGICAL IMPACT OF TRAUMA EXPOSURE ON THE HELPER

The discovery of mirror neurons in the 1990s at the University of Parma helped to shed light on what happens when people have a shared experience. Researchers found that the shared experiences individuals have with one another are inextricably linked (Iacoboni, 2008). It turns out that when people see each other, their brains build a detailed simulation of what they are seeing, including the motor components. It is as though they see themselves as the person they are watching for a split second. The brain truly tries to feel what the other person is feeling, and it interprets what is being seen as a shared experience with others. What this means in practical terms is that "in other people, we see ourselves" (Iacoboni, 2008, p.134).

Iacoboni (2008) further writes,

> Our mirror neurons fire when we see others expressing their emotions, as if we were making those facial expressions ourselves. By means of this firing, the neurons also send signals to emotional brain centers in the limbic system to make us feel what other people feel. (p. 119)

The significance of this for helpers is that when the helper is listening, engaging, or literally helping an individual through a crisis, their body and mirror neuron system is picking up on the individual's nonverbal and verbal cues, which are directly linked to what is happening inside of the individual's nervous system. These cues support the helper in feeling what the person being helped is feeling. For example, as an individual shares and describes the specific details of a traumatic event, their body will begin to demonstrate fear, overwhelm, helplessness, or other emotions that they are experiencing as they remember the event. As the helper observes, listens, and interacts, somatic shifts will emerge inside of the helper supporting the helper to feel what it is like inside of the individual. This means that the helper will feel the effects of the trauma exposure, whether they want to or not. This puts helpers in an incredibly vulnerable position—in order to be of service to others, they must also learn how to navigate the inevitable trauma activation that occurs inside of them. Without this, the helper can internalize these emotional experiences as though they had personally experienced them.

Words such as compassion fatigue, vicarious trauma, or secondary traumatization (American Counseling Association, 2011; Figley, 2002) have been used to describe the emotional impact of exposure when helping others vicariously process their traumatic experiences. It refers to the emotional residue of exposure to traumatic stories and experiences of others through work while witnessing fear, pain, and terror that others have experienced (American Counseling Association, 2011). For this chapter, the term secondary traumatization will be highlighted.

In addition to the somatic shifts that occur in the moment of helping, other symptoms such as intrusive images, nightmares, and high states of nervous system dysregulation are also common (American Counseling Association, 2011). Experiences such as these can lead to increased agitation, anxiety and depression, emotional numbing, and hypervigilance. These secondary traumatization symptoms can develop over time or can develop from a single case of exposure. The impact greatly depends on how much support the helper receives, how emotionally resourced the helper is, and the degree to which the trauma exposure activates the helper's own trauma history. How direct the contact is with the trauma or trauma victims themselves and the level of exposure to stories, photos, graphic explanations, environments and other details of the traumatic events also influence the impact.

Helpers often enter helping professions because they want to be of service to others. However, being in a position that requires them to feel some degree of trauma activation in their own body alongside the person they are helping can, over time, influence the helper's perception of themselves and the world around them. The helper may end up not feeling safe, feeling more cynical, and feeling more helpless and hopeless (American Counseling Association, 2011; Stamm et al., 2002), ultimately resulting in the helper no longer wanting to or no longer being able to be a helper. Studies also suggest that ongoing trauma exposure can lead to an increase in alcohol and drug use, as well as physical illness (Giordano, 2021; Holmes et al., 2021).

It is important to note that each time the helper is exposed to trauma, cortisol is produced in the body, and over time, the helper can begin to adapt to these elevated cortisol levels (Beckley-Forest & Monaco, 2020). As this occurs, the helper can lose the ability to respond to stress adaptively. They may acquire a "new normal" in terms of their active level of arousal contributing to many of the symptoms of secondary traumatization. The body also begins to monitor for safety cues more frequently. In other words, in the absence of a genuine external threat, the helper unconsciously activates the fear reaction linking the fear to the original trauma. This process is known as neurosensitization (Scaer, 2012).

## IMPACT OF HELPER'S SECONDARY TRAUMATIZATION ON PERSON BEING HELPED

In order to integrate the impact of trauma, an individual must be able to safely and mindfully move toward the associated thoughts, feelings, and body sensations, which often require support from a helper (Dion, 2018). As an individual is retelling and thus reliving the trauma, the associated feelings and need for safety will naturally surface. It is in these moments that the individual will need support from the helper. They will, in a sense, attempt to borrow the helper's regulatory capacity (Dion, 2018) or in other words, seek to feel grounded and safe in the helper's presence. Part of what the helpers are offering to the individual in need during these moments is co-regulation. This provides support for the individual to move toward their uncomfortable thoughts, feelings, and body sensations in order to integrate the impact and create an internalized sense of safety (Schore, 2003, 2019).

The helper must be able to be present with not only the individual's activation but also their own in order to do this. They must be able to hold the intensity without getting lost in it; separating out their own trauma history from the individual's trauma they are supporting in the moment. This requires active self-regulation on the part of the helper, which will be explored through the lens of Polyvagal Theory (Dana, 2023; Porges, 2011, 2021) later in this chapter.

When a helper is experiencing symptoms of secondary trauma, this process becomes increasingly more complicated as the helper becomes limited in their ability to be with the emotional intensity of what is arising internally, and thus their ability to co-regulate decreases. As a result, the helper becomes more susceptible to misattunement, projecting their assumptions about the experience of the trauma onto the individual they are trying to help, increased emotional flooding, and their own protective patterns emerging. In these moments, the individual being helped can feel missed, not seen, not heard, and in some cases experience a compounding effect to their trauma.

## CASE EXAMPLE

Matthew sits down across from Jonathan, his therapist, and begins to share what happened. When Matthew was seven years old, he was sexually abused by his grandfather. Mathew is now an adult and for the first time is ready to share the details of his story. As Jonathan attentively listens to Matthew's story, he begins to notice that his stomach is tightening and that there is a giant lump in his throat. He feels incredibly sad inside and has the urge to withdraw. Although he has been trained to listen and witness his client's hard stories, each one carries with it its own pain. In each instance, Jonathan is asked to be with his client in that pain. Later that night, Jonathan can't stop thinking about Matthew as a seven-year-old boy and what happened to him. As he does, he feels the same tightening in his stomach, lump in his throat, and sadness. Over the next few weeks, Jonathan notices that he feels more sensitive and a bit more withdrawn.

In the case of Matthew, imagining his client as a young boy and the experience he went through turned into intrusive thoughts in the night and days following the session. With each intrusive thought also came dysregulation in his own physiology experienced as tightening in his stomach and lumps in his throat, followed by sadness and a desire to withdraw. This was the same somatic activation that he experienced as he was listening to his client's story during the session, likely imagining what it was like being his client during the traumatic event. The impact of hearing this story stayed with him for several weeks resulting in further emotional withdrawal and feeling more emotionally sensitive. From the perspective of Interpersonal Neurobiology, this can be understood as his window of tolerance (capacity to hold the intensity) became smaller (Siegel, 2010).

During the next session with Matthew, Jonathan noticed that each time he looked at Matthew, he could not help but think of the pain of the seven-year-old boy. As Matthew continued to share more of the story, Jonathan's sadness continued to grow, making it difficult for him to stay present with Matthew. What Jonathan was not consciously aware of was that although he was not sexually abused, he did have his own childhood experiences where he felt helpless. These past unresolved experiences were being triggered in his session with his client. Through this experience, his past protective pattern of emotionally withdrawing was activated. In the therapy session, this translated into his client feeling less attuned to him and a bit more emotionally guarded. Sensing Jonathan's emotional withdrawal, Matthew intuitively stopped sharing as many details of his story.

This example is not uncommon when a helper's unresolved trauma is aroused. In these moments, the helper will use whatever tools and protective patterns that are available in an effort to self-govern, including attempts to move away from content that activates specific bodily sensations and emotions. This moving away can look like denying the existence of the sensations or emotions or shutting them down in some manner. Behaviors such as changing the topic, engaging in problem-solving strategies, staying task-oriented, and compartmentalization, are common coping strategies. When

Jonathan felt the sensations in his body, he tried to move away from them in order to deal with the intensity. Another normal response when the helper cannot self-govern is to become emotionally overwhelmed, which can translate into dissociation or high levels of dysregulation within the autonomic nervous system.

There is a common misconception that helpers would not or do not get triggered by their own unresolved trauma experiences and that activation can be avoided. Interpersonal Neurobiology informs us that although these moments are inevitable, the person being helped can still be impacted when they do occur. It is in these moments that the helper's ability to be present in the activation and self-regulate becomes paramount, so that they do not direct the person being helped away from their own experience of what they are trying to process (Beckley-Forest & Monaco, 2020). It also means that if an attachment ruptures and mis-attunement does occur with the person being helped, it is important to come back and do repair to reestablish a neuroception of safety (Porges, 2021; Schore, 2019).

When helpers are not willing or able to become aware of what is happening inside of themselves and regulate through it, they increase the likelihood of merging with the person they are trying to help. They also increase the possibility of moving emotionally too far away from them and moving the person also away from what they are trying to emotionally process. The result is that both the helper and the person being helped have a higher probability of not integrating the impact of the trauma exposure.

Sieff (2015) describes the importance of a therapist's ability to self-regulate during these moments in the following way: "When a therapist's wounds are hit, can she regulate her own bodily based emotions and shame dynamics well enough to be able to stay connected to her patient? Can the therapist tolerate what is happening in her own body when it mirrors her patient's terror, rage and physiological hyperarousal. . . . Herein lies the art of psychotherapy" (p. 132). These same questions can be applied to all helpers. To reiterate, a helper's own activation is unavoidable. What the helper does or does not do in response is the key to being able to continue to help the individual integrate their trauma.


## HELPING THE HELPER

Although it is inevitable that the helper will be impacted in some way by trauma exposure, there is much that can be done to mitigate the effects and to decrease the risks of secondary traumatization. Much of the literature on this topic addresses what can be done after the trauma exposure occurs and when there is ongoing exposure. These include, but are not limited to the following:

1. Get support—Receiving support is incredibly important as holding onto the trauma alone can compound the trauma. Helpers need helpers to help them process, make sense of, normalize, and integrate their experiences. They need others to help them find their own internal sense of safety, much like the helper is doing for those they are helping.

2. Develop a self-care strategy—For many helpers, they are more inclined to help others than help themselves, and thus their own self-care can be ignored. It is important that each helper discovers for themselves what is needed as each person is different. What might feel like self-care to one individual may not feel like self-care to another. Ideas include exercise, journaling, creating, singing, dancing, massage, and meditation. Self-care also includes taking time off, having quiet time, and spending time connecting with others.

3. Know limits and set boundaries—It is common for helpers to overextend themselves, pushing themselves outside their windows of tolerance, thereby increasing the effect of the trauma exposure. Learning to notice when boundaries need to be set and when limits need to be addressed is critical for mitigating secondary traumatization.

4. Refuel—Taking time to engage in activities that feel fulfilling not only helps the body but also helps combat the cynicism and mental exhaustion that can start to set in with ongoing trauma exposure. Engaging in activities that refuel can remind the helper that there is still hope, joy, goodness, and inspiration in the world.

In addition to the above, it turns out that support for secondary traumatization no longer needs to only occur after the exposure but can also occur *in the moment* of the exposure itself—helping both the helper and the person being helped.

In 2011, Dr. Stephen Porges introduced the Polyvagal Theory into the field of Interpersonal Neurobiology bringing new insight and understanding of the nervous system and the importance of having a felt sense of safety for trauma integration. These new insights offer new possibilities for helpers as they navigate the complexities of trauma exposure. At its core, Polyvagal Theory is about safety. It is about learning how to access a ventral vagal response in the midst of the sympathetic and dorsal parasympathetic protective responses of the autonomic nervous system. It is the activation of the ventral vagal response that contributes to the ability to modulate the activation of these protective responses helping create what is referred to as a "neuroception of safety" (Porges, 2011, 2021).

For further explanation, when an individual experiences something challenging, their autonomic nervous system is designed to respond for protection. Depending on whether or not the individual perceives they can do something about the situation influences whether their system revs up into a sympathetic flight/fight response to take on the challenge or goes into a dorsal parasympathetic response shutting down and moving toward immobilization for protection. These responses are all part of the activation that occurs during a traumatic situation and as previously described, will also naturally be relived *together* as the person being helped is retelling, remembering (consciously or unconsciously), and playing out their traumatic memories.

It is worth mentioning that the intensity of these protective responses is likely to increase when the helper is experiencing the same trauma as those actively needing help. This was the experience of many front-line workers during the COVID-19 pandemic and that of many first responders in other times of crisis. This shared experience adds another complexity to being a helper. In these situations, helpers are at an even higher risk of their own emotional flooding and overwhelm as the trauma unfolds in real time. In these scenarios, the primary task for the helper is to create a neuroception of safety within themselves first and then for the person they are trying to help, so that they do not compound the trauma they are both already experiencing. Sometimes this means addressing basic needs to create physical safety before being able to create emotional safety.

When the body naturally moves into flight/fight or starts to shut down into immobilization, the helper's ability to access their own ventral vagal response and bring in a neuroception of safety is paramount. The helper's ability to do this is the key to mitigating the effects of trauma exposure and experiencing symptoms of secondary traumatization. The ventral vagal system helps an individual to be able to modulate the activation of the protective responses. Another term that is often used to describe this process is *regulation*. There is a common misconception about regulation that might impair a helper's ability to help others through self-regulation and co-regulation. The common misconception is that regulation equals calm. When the body is in a protective reaction, becoming calm is incredibly challenging as the body is activated for a reason, not to mention if what is needed in the moment is to run or move for safety, becoming calm may not be the best strategy. Regulation has more to do with the ability to mindfully connect to oneself (Dion, 2018) in the midst of the activation in order to decide what the body needs at the moment to modulate the intensity. Experiencing what is going on within the body while listening, engaging, or helping someone through trauma is unpleasant, but it is necessary to appropriately attune to the experience of the person being helped. One of the most crucial abilities helpers need to acquire is the ability to maintain a relationship with their bodies and expand their capacity to feel while remaining connected to themselves.The following are ways to access the ventral vagal response, mindfully connect to oneself, and begin to create a neuroception of safety in the midst of trauma exposure:

1. Mindfully Breathe—When we move into sympathetic arousal or dorsal parasympathetic collapse, our breathing patterns change. Mindfully taking longer inhalations or exhalations, depending on what the body needs, is a helpful way to connect and find an internal anchor.
2. Move your body—When the body becomes activated, it revs up or shuts down. Moving the body (e.g., walking, tapping feet back and forth, squeezing arms, shaking hands, and stretching) helps the helper stay connected and in their window of tolerance.
3. Name your experience out loud—"Name it to tame it" was a phrase coined by Dr. Daniel Siegel and explains how naming an internal experience out loud helps settle the activation in the nervous system.
4. Ask for help—Remembering that sometimes the intensity is just too much and that it is ok to ask to pause and/or ask for help.

In the case example of Jonathan, while he was listening to his client tell his story and he noticed his stomach tightening and the lump in his throat, he could have taken some mindful breaths to help himself ground or move his body to help him be with the uncomfortable sensations instead of falling back on his old protective pattern of withdrawing. Doing so would have also helped Matthew continue to feel Jonathan's presence and regulatory capacity as he was telling his story, helping him feel safe enough to keep going toward what felt uncomfortable for integration. It would have potentially given Jonathan insight into Matthew's experience, which could have supported further connection. Jonathan continuing to mindfully *be with himself* while tracking his own activation (accessing his ventral vagal response in the midst of his nervous system dysregulation) likely would have also had a helpful impact on the symptoms of vicarious trauma that he later experienced.

As the helper feels the inevitable somatic shifts occurring inside as they help, they simultaneously become aware of the activation while also accessing their own ventral state, which allows a neuroception of safety to form within. This process can be further understood as being both regulated and dysregulated at the same time as the intensity arises (Dion, 2018). The very act of bringing in a sense of safety through connecting with the self is what allows the helper to think a bit more clearly, feel a bit more grounded, stay connected to their body, and integrate the impact of the trauma exposure. The helper can then hold both the felt experience of the person being helped, as well as what is happening inside of them while not being swept up in intensity. The result is the helper is able to attune, be present, think more clearly, and respond instead of reacting. From this state of regulation, the helper is able to co-regulate the person they are trying to help, supporting them to also find a felt sense of safety so that they can move toward their own uncomfortable thoughts, feelings, and body sensations as they navigate the impact of their trauma.

## CONCLUSION

Helpers are extraordinary individuals who dedicate their lives to being of service to others, but not without risk. Ongoing trauma exposure places these individuals in highly susceptible positions for developing symptoms of secondary traumatization. For this reason, helpers must become aware of the unavoidable impact of trauma exposure, understand the signs of secondary traumatization, and most importantly, learn what to do to minimize the impact and integrate their experiences. Finding support and practicing self-care is paramount, but with new understandings from Polyvagal Theory and Interpersonal Neurobiology, helpers are now equipped with further knowledge of the need to regulate in the midst of the activation of the exposure, along with doing what they can for secondary traumatization prevention outside of the exposure. In both cases, the primary goal for the helper is to create a neuroception of safety within themselves, in order to co-regulate with the person, they are trying to help toward their own internal sense of safety and ultimate integration of the trauma.

## REFERENCES

American Counseling Association (2011). Fact Sheet #9: Vicarious trauma. https://www.counseling.org/sub/dmh/Fact%20Sheet%209%20-%20Vicarious%20Traum.pdf

Center for Disease Control (2021). Adverse Childhood Experiences—ACEs. https://www.cdc.gov/vitalsigns/aces/index.html

Beckley-Forest, A., & Monaco, A. (2020). *EMDR with children in the play therapy room: An integrated approach.* Springer Publishing.

Dana, D. (2023). *Polyvagal practices: Anchoring the self in safety.* Norton Publishing.

Dion, L. (2018). *Aggression in play therapy: A neurobiological approach for integrating intensity.* Norton Publishing.

Figley, C. (2002). Compassion fatigue: Psychotherapists chronic lack of self-care. *Journal of Clinical Psychology/In Session, 58*(11), 1433–1441.

Giordano, A. (2021). *Why trauma can lead to addiction.* Psychology Today. https://www.psychologytoday.com/us/blog/understanding-addiction/202109/why-trauma-can-lead-addiction#

Holmes, M. R., Rentrope, C. R., Korsch-Williams, A., & King, J. A. (2021). Impact of COVID-19 pandemic on posttraumatic stress, grief, burnout, and secondary trauma of social workers in the United States. *National Library of Medicine.* https://www.ncbi.nlm.nih.gov/pmc/articles/PMC7922703/

Iacoboni, M. (2008). *Mirroring people: The new science of how we connect with others.* Farrar, Straus and Giroux.

Porges, S. W. (2011). *The Polyvagal Theory: Neurophysiological foundations of emotions, attachment, communication, self-regulation.* Norton.

Porges, S. W. (2021). *Polyvagal safety: Attachment. communication, self-regulation.* Norton.

Scaer, R. (2012). *8 Keys to Brain-Body Balance.* Norton.

Schore, A. N. (2003). *Affect regulation and the repair of the self.* Norton.

Schore, A. N. (2019). *Right brain psychotherapy.* Norton.

Sieff, D. F. (2015). *Understanding and healing emotional trauma: Conversations with pioneering clinicians and researchers.* Routledge.

Siegel, D. J. (Ed.) (2010). *The mindful therapist: A clinician's guide to mindsight and neural integration.* Norton.

Siegel, D. J. (2020). *The developing mind, third edition: How relationships and the brain interact to shape who we are.* Guilford Press.

Stamm, B.H., Varra, E.M., Pearlman, L.A., & Giller, E. (2002) *The helper's power to heal and to be hurt—or helped—by trying.* Washington, DC: Register Report: A Publication of the National Register of Health Service Providers in Psychology.

# FUTURE IMPLICATIONS AND PROGRESSIVE SUPPORTS OF TRAUMA IMPACTS

## CHAPTER FOURTEEN

# A Process-Oriented and Multilayered Approach to the Global Impacts of Trauma

CLAUDIO MOCHI and ISABELLA CASSINA

## TRAUMATIC EVENTS: WHAT WE DO NOT SEE

Research shows that in spite of adversity, there are protective and well-being factors such as the power of human connection and play, which allow one to create safety and opportunities for growth even in the most complex situations (MacFarlane, 1987; Masten & Narayan, 2011; Perry, 2007). While a traumatic event may induce horror, helplessness, and despair, an individual's access to relationships and a break from trauma via play allows one to master and process complex events; to invent, compensate, and develop skills useful in overcoming challenging situations (Bettelheim, 1987; Ginsburg, 2007; Schaefer & Drewes, 2014). Play is a tool for cultivating resilience by strengthening neural circuits that help optimize the regulation of the physiological states and move rapidly from a condition of activation to one of calm (Porges, 2021). Furthermore, the attitude of carers offers a powerful protective factor even in the face of the most overwhelming circumstances. Mochi (2022) proposed that adults are dispensers of safety for young children. Masten and Narayan (2011) furthered, "the buffering effect of proximity to parents and other attachment figures for children in the midst of terrifying

*Trauma Impacts: The Repercussions of Individual and Collective Trauma*, First Edition.
Edited by Jessica Stone, Robert J. Grant, and Clair Mellenthin.
© 2024 John Wiley & Sons, Inc. Published 2024 by John Wiley & Sons, Inc.

experiences is one of the most enduring findings in the literature on war and other life-threatening disasters" (p. 3).

Resilience can be exercised and is certainly nurtured by many interactions especially if they combine the presence of social support, a thoughtful caregiver, and the possibility of playing. However, the pathway to endure or recover from a variety of difficulties is complex and influenced by many elements that are not easily observable or predictable, and so much of it cannot be understood in the immediate aftermath of a crisis. It is not simple to grasp what an individual is missing, how onerous the daily struggle of adults and children is, and how far the threshold of endurance is before their coping capacities are exceeded and the situation becomes unbearable. Nor is the cascade of events that can follow a given situation predictable. Adaptation to traumatic circumstances is a "dynamic process involving multiple interacting systems within the individual organism and many interactions of the individual with complex and changing contexts" (Masten & Narayan, 2011, p. 4).

Different studies (Masten & Narayan, 2011; Perry, 2007; Schore, 2019) argue that exposure to challenges of moderate intensity and duration can help make the body increasingly adept at handling difficult situations; however, everyone has limits. Several authors (Perry et al., 1995; Sameroff et al., 1987; Shore, 1997) underline that chronic levels of stress and scarcity of learning opportunities can affect a child's development and lifetime possibilities. Moreover, "cumulative effects from multiple risk factors increase the probability that development will be compromised" (Sameroff et al., 1987, p. 343).

This dynamic acquires even more meaning when supported by the avalanche metaphor (Cassina, 2023). Using the symbolism of an avalanche, risk factors build upon one another, just like the layers of snow on a mountain. The deposit of each layer of snow following a storm makes the entire structure unstable and susceptible to failure. As the accumulation of risk grows, so does the potential power for destruction. Once an avalanche begins to cascade down the mountain, building in intensity, nothing can stop the powerful destruction from taking place. As Masten and Narayan (2011) state, the impact of stressful events beyond a certain threshold tends to expand from one domain to another; the same thing happens when a mass of snow in its descent accumulates further material and destructive power.

Just as a large avalanche cannot be stopped by a small plain, circumstances of high psychosocial distress and conditions of trauma cannot be recovered by sporadic, albeit enjoyable, activities. In order to slow down, stop an avalanche, and mitigate its devastating effects, it is necessary for the entire community to take action with multiple interventions: managing the initial impact, restoring the starting conditions when appropriate, reinforcing the context as a whole, and defining a prevention plan. This is one of the main

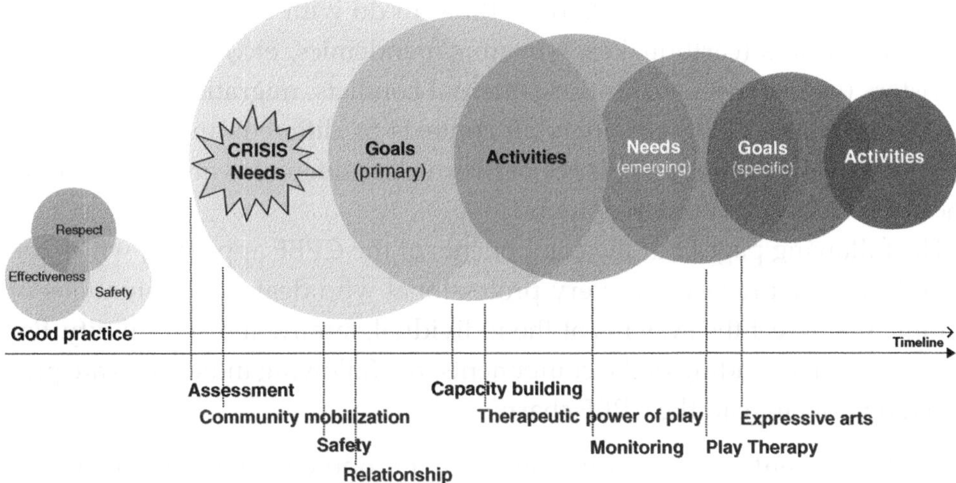


**Figure 14.1** The approach "Coping with the present while building for the future" (CPBF). Reproduced with permission Isabella Cassina & Claudio Mochi (2023), Routledge/ Taylor & Francis.

reasons underlying the approach "Coping with the present while building for the future" (CPBF) (Cassina & Mochi, 2023) illustrated in Figure 14.1, also referred to as "CPBF chart."

The difficulties and the multiplication of vulnerability factors in the face of limited possibilities for recovery leave a huge mark and require expanding the boundaries of the "serene oases" and multiplying the possibilities for healthy growth and well-being.

## COPING WITH THE PRESENT WHILE BUILDING FOR THE FUTURE

The approach CPBF developed through international field practice in collaboration with a multitude of local actors. The corresponding chart (Figure 14.1) represents the result of a theoretical synthesis and should be considered as the authors' MAP (My Awareness Process) (Mochi, 2022).

A MAP is the awareness process and knowledge that each professional or organisation should bring with them as they move into unknown critical scenarios. A MAP assists to sustain partners and local professionals in gaining a sense of safety, orientation, and understanding in confusing or dangerous times. A MAP includes all necessary elements that support the co-construction of the entire crisis intervention. (Cassina & Mochi, 2023, p. 13)

Although the CPBF approach originates from work in crisis scenarios, its underlying principles can be generalized to contexts of high vulnerability and complexity that have little or nothing to do with crises in the sense of natural disasters (earthquakes, tsunamis, pandemics, etc.) or human-made disasters (wars between countries, internal conflicts, migration, etc.). This is possible because CPBF considers all contexts as different and unique, and emphasizes the need for a balance between clear references and flexibility in the co-construction of interventions.

The following pages outline components of the CPBF approach, which are useful in daily practice for every professional who deals with situations of trauma that affect the systems of the individual, family, and community. For a clearer understanding of the components, the following indications are provided on how to read the CPBF chart:

1. The elements/actions are arranged in chronological order from left to right. This means that some actions lay the foundations for subsequent ones to take place. For example, it is not desirable to conduct play therapy sessions with a child without first having an overview of their context as clear as possible, and without having established a trusting relationship, at least with their caregiver(s) or other reference adult(s).

2. The timing for moving from one element/action to another is flexible, depends on a number of context variables, and should not be rushed. For example, the timeframe for achieving the primary goals (including safety and relationship) depends on the starting conditions. If we are in a context where a war is taking place and/or a natural disaster has recently occurred, the timeframe will inevitably be longer than in circumstances that, although traumatic, have less or no devastating effect on the community as a whole.

3. Moving on to the next element/action does not mean that the previous one is fully completed. For example, the feeling of safety is not easily and permanently achieved. This must be a constant concern for the therapist or disaster worker throughout the duration of the intervention. The same applies to the needs assessment, which is carried out at the beginning, and also repeated regularly.

4. In accordance with the mission to cope with the present and build for the future, the CPBF chart follows the "need-goal-activity" (N-G-A) pattern. This pattern emphasizes the importance of detecting existing needs, defining corresponding goals, and promoting them through a series of activities. These activities will be fundamental for detecting future needs for which new goals and activities will be established. What is done today is the foundation for what will be done in the future to ensure effectiveness and sustainability.

CASE EXAMPLE

Mila and Beyond

Mila was an eight-year-old child of Roma ethnicity who moved from Kosovo with her family because of the war in the former Yugoslavia. There was very little information about her early years. Her grandparents told us that they had started looking after her at some point after her parents had abandoned her. They did not have a permanent home for a long time, but for the last two years, they had been living in shacks near one of the Collective Centres (facilities used to accommodate the displaced population), which were part of a long-standing psychosocial project. Mila's grandparents contacted us during one of our monitoring visits.

In her class, Mila was the only child with wheat-colored hair. She seemed shy and never participated in activities. Her grandparents had been repeatedly urged by the teachers to enroll her in a school for children with special needs. Mila could barely read and was considered very behind her peers. When we visited her at school, she was sitting alone behind a small desk at the back of the class. The teachers would tell us: "She is very stubborn. . .," "She has an oppositional disorder. . . and a learning disorder!," "She doesn't have any disorder. . . She is just insolent!." Everyone at school had a different opinion, but they all agreed that Mila was distracting and slowing down her classmates and wanted to find another placement for her.

Even though Mila was hearing impaired, she had been seated at the back of the classroom from where she heard nothing of what was going on. The treatment and marginalization by the teachers seemed to justify marginalization by her classmates as well. She had no friends, and even at the Roma camp, she remained alone most of the time, confined to her grandparents' living spaces. She was relieved to skip school for whatever reason, including helping with household management. Her story was complex, with many gray areas and uncertainties. In addition to neglect and parental abandonment, we could not exclude that Mila had experienced further traumatic events. The intervention for her healthy growth and well-being had to include a multitude of actions and actors in the field.

THE GROUNDING PHASE

Adverse events can create conditions of vulnerability, widespread symptomatology, chronic psychopathology, and also an impact on future generations (Masten & Cicchetti, 2010; Masten & Narayan, 2011; van der Kolk, 2014; Yehuda et al., 2007). The story of Mila is a good example of the complexity that characterizes many situations around the world. Behind the behavior labeled insolence, much more was happening, including the weight of unmet needs and possible traumatic events. We consider it important to emphasize that the reasoning we are going to make regarding the feeling of safety is not limited to children like Mila but is applicable to people of all age groups. Specifically, in crisis contexts, the entire population is subject to prolonged conditions of extreme vulnerability: children, caregivers, professionals, helpers, and adults in general.

A single event has the power to change the course of a life, let alone a chronic multitude of adverse events experienced. The more chronic or complex the trauma experience is, the higher the possibility of developing long-term pathologies. The combination of post-traumatic symptomatology and exposure to adverse events predisposes to the development of a range of other difficulties such as "eating disorders, depression, suicidal behaviour, anxiety, alcoholism, violent behaviour, mood disorders, etc." (Perry, 2007, p. 8), and significant physical problems in adulthood, including "heart disease, cancer, chronic lung disease, and various risk behaviours" (Perry, 2007, p. 8). The traumatic event may affect multiple spheres of life and have repercussions over the years, especially if social support is lacking.

One of the consequences of trauma is that it retunes the autonomic nervous system from calmness and spontaneous social engagement to defense, thus interfering with the ability to socially engage, communicate, and connect. To use an image, it is as if people in the aftermath of multiple threatening events surround themselves with high, thick walls for protection, thereby limiting involvement with the outside world. Traumatic events can push a defensive state to become a permanent state and transform the refuge within the walls, or what we love to depict as a "castle", from a temporary shelter to a habitual residence, causing serious impairment of the individual's possibilities and well-being. Indeed, only by leaving the castle and thus regaining a basic level of safety can health, growth, and restoration be achieved.

In this regard, the Polyvagal Theory (Porges, 2015, 2017, 2021) highlights several important aspects. The perception of danger that triggers the defensive reaction occurs below one's level of awareness through the neural process called "neuroception." Overcoming a defensive state occurs through two pathways, one of which is passive and happens outside of conscious awareness, while the other is active and requires voluntary behavior. The recovery of an initial state of safety depends on the passive pathway to access and use the active one. Referring to our castle metaphor, the individual does not choose to enter the castle and cannot be forced out either. We cannot force a condition of safety, and consequently, it may also be counterproductive to impose one's own help. It would be like trying to scale castle fortifications or to breach them. This would either lead the individual to fortify their defenses or surrender completely. On the contrary, it is the constant and unconscious perception of safety cues from the surroundings (passive pathway) that can push one to start looking outside the castle walls. Any intervention in crisis contexts should send safety messages that progressively stimulate the lowering of defenses and encourage connection.

Groundwork is the set of operations that makes it possible for people to regain a sense of safety and build a relationship of trust with the professional(s). As stated above, professionals need to take into account individual's layers of defensiveness while being present outside the castle walls, at a distance that respects time and space but is also easily accessible, ready to listen, and be supportive. Groundwork is also necessary for professionals to assess the context, needs, and resources in order to co-construct a set of interconnected actions that can support individuals, families, and communities. A fundamental initial component of the CPBF approach is to create the conditions that allow the individual to step outside the castle walls. Only when the person feels safe enough to venture around, will it be possible to initiate an active process that leads through different stages to health, growth, and restoration.

## THE SAFEST POSSIBLE ENVIRONMENT

Complicated contexts require a breadth of vision and a starting point. Our starting point is always inspired by the principles governing "good practice" (Cassina & Mochi, 2023; Mochi, 2022). As indicated on the left side of the CPBF chart, good practice is the combination of respect, effectiveness, and safety through the power of connection. Starting from there, the minimum goal is the creation of the Safest Possible Environment (SaPE) (Mochi & Cassina, 2024) since "we need a sense of safety to support health, growth and restoration" (Porges, 2015, p. 115). Any intervention should aim at maximizing the chances to stimulate a feeling of safety. A key factor is recognizing, together with the importance of safety, that change is easier when it is stably nurtured by the widest possible number of sources. The direct consequence implies a multiplicity of interventions, both inside and outside the therapy room.

Mila needed specialized treatment inside the playroom, but she also needed daily support outside the playroom starting with feeling safer at school and in her life context. A first step in cooperation with local educators and social workers was to make the teachers aware of the child's uncertain living conditions, suggest how her behavior could be the result of possible traumatic events, and to move Mila to a desk in the front row so that she could better hear what was happening during the lessons. "Schools are in a unique position to provide children with resources such as a safe context, structure, and guidance, co-regulation, learning material, and the stimulation of a child's emerging abilities" (Mochi & Stagnitti, 2023, p. 104). When this potential is not fully utilized, it is worth taking action to stimulate change.

## A MULTILAYERED APPROACH

In contexts characterized by traumatic events, the careful management of time and space is extremely relevant. Professionals are expected not only to promptly provide responses to the most pressing needs in the field but also to create the necessary conditions for connection and understanding of local dynamics. It is important to offer structure and predictability but also to provide space for initiative and the natural local recovery process. Preestablished and standardized programs, lack of involvement of local resources, and specialized interventions carried out prematurely can fail to capture the complexity of needs and even be counterproductive. In contrast, groundwork makes possible effective and sustainable interventions aimed at (a) involvement, (b) empowerment, and (c) treatment of the most complex issues.

Figure 14.2 is a synthesis of a more articulated chart that originally appeared in the book "Beyond the Clouds" (Mochi, 2022), an autoethnographic research that explores the good practices in crisis settings. The chart represents the stages of a crisis intervention focusing on the role of play coherently with the CPBF approach. The triangle shape (a trend

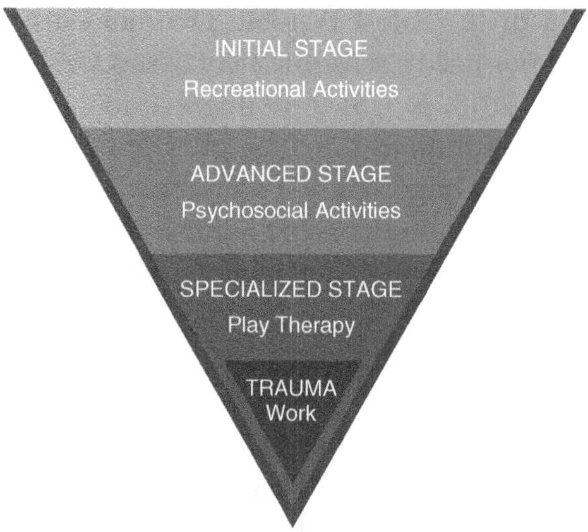


**Figure 14.2**  The stages of a crisis intervention: focusing on trauma.

represented in the CPBF chart with six circles of progressively smaller size), represents the authors' recommendation to involve more people in the initial stage of the intervention and gradually decrease it as the intervention becomes more specialized.

> In the initial stage, recreational activities can be implemented to involve as many people as possible. In the advanced stage, psychosocial activities are directed to selected groups of children. In the specialised stage, play therapy interventions involve a small number of children and families who are in need of this kind of involvement. (Cassina & Mochi, 2023, p. 21)

Unlike the original chart, Figure 14.2 graphically highlights the positioning of trauma work. As anticipated, working on trauma without having laid the groundwork poses limitations, including the risk of intervening inappropriately and less effectively for the individual, creating unpleasant and confusing dynamics for family and colleagues, and ignoring important cultural aspects should our intervention take place abroad. That said, a focus on trauma is placed from the very beginning (the darker color referring to "trauma work" forms the background to the whole triangle). Recreational activities can precisely be the time and context to start identifying the need for trauma-related intervention through observation, sharing, and collecting information. However, since prolonged and severe trauma situations can only worsen the individual's condition (Masten & Narayan, 2011; Perry, 2007; van der Kolk, 2014), the start of specific treatments can be expected relatively quickly.

Mila's referral came to us in a context that was not only prepared for a multilayered intervention, but in which work in Collective Centres had already begun years before and boasted the collaboration of a local network of professionals and parents. Mila's school was not yet officially involved in the project but was aware of it, her grandparents knew us by sight and had heard about us from other caregivers. The triggering of a specialized intervention was therefore quick and timely in relation to the report received. With the grandparents' consent, Mila started an individual therapy process in which play therapy methodologies were employed by trained and supervised local mental health professionals. In child-centered play therapy sessions (VanFleet et al., 2010), Mila's prevalent play themes were good versus bad and competence. In early sessions, she repeatedly won at games such as darts and basketball. Afterward, she experimented with building and repairing various objects and impersonated a doctor who had the power to decide the fate of those around her. Her pretend play was increasingly complex. Very soon Mila began to participate in playgroups and to benefit from individual school support, thanks to the involvement of volunteer professionals.

## INVOLVING CAREGIVERS

Mila's grandparents allowed the child to attend extracurricular activities and were willing to listen to occasional feedback, but unfortunately, it was not possible to involve them more in the child's play therapy process or other activities dedicated to caregivers. This does not mean that other reference adults did not appear in her life. Mila was no longer the child alone at the back of the class. She had an increasing number of people at her side including her play therapist, support teacher at school, and educators during extracurricular activities. These people multiplied her experiences of safety, unconditional acceptance, and development of skills.

The involvement of caregivers and other reference adults is fundamental to the intervention and follows the considerations and guidelines proposed so far. Caregivers should also feel safe, have the chance to develop awareness of the situation, enhance their own resources and capabilities, and acquire or consolidate the ability to actively manage their world. These possibilities ought to be promoted from as many sources as possible through groundwork and a multilayered intervention. In our international fieldwork, for instance, we developed the following:

- *Informal spaces* for listening and sharing while drinking a cup of tea or coffee. This would allow caregivers to have a first spatial–temporal reference point, begin to have a hint of routine again, and, over time, feeling increasingly comfortable and safe. As explained by Porges (2015, 2017, 2021), this last aspect implies the practitioner's use of a prosodic voice, warm and welcoming facial expressions, and gestures of accessibility as well as a specific structuring of the spaces, which must be welcoming, possibly bright, spacious, isolated from noise, guarantee privacy, include cozy seating, the possibility of movement, expressive, and creative materials to become familiar with.

- *Recreational and informative activities* determined according to the needs, interests, and culture of the specific group. These activities make it possible to enhance personal resources, acquire new insights, connect regularly with others in similar situations, and experience enjoyable moments in a predictable way. The activities should be the result of co-construction with the persons involved. In Pakistan, for example, a group of female caregivers organized sewing and cooking sessions; in India, young fathers developed a music workshop; and in Iran, mothers were interested in understanding trauma and learning how to deal with children's tantrums.

- *Psychosocial activities* including the possibility of group meetings that apply playful and creative modalities. Indeed, play and the expressive arts have transformative and healing powers that can be applied to address challenges. Psychosocial activities led by trained professionals can guide caregivers in using creative modalities to feel an active part in developing their own solutions. "The fulfilment of experiencing one's own creativity through [play and] art-making lends courage and motivation to the task of confronting and releasing destructive life experiences" (Halprin, 1999, p. 137).

- *Psychotherapy* possibly through the expressive arts such as movement, music, image-making, performance, writing, play, and imagination (Levine, 2019; Malchiodi, 2020). Some caregivers and other reference adults facing critical contexts may need specialized care for the treatment of major psychological disorders and trauma. This is a possibility that should always be considered and provided, regardless of the magnitude of the crisis or the moment. Indeed, this need may be manifested in the short or long term.

We do not want to deny that involving caregivers is as important as it is difficult. In contexts of high vulnerability, the adult population is faced with a large number of challenges and responsibilities that often make the castle walls and fortifications particularly tall and armored. That said, it is always worth a try.

## CONCLUSION

Trauma is a desolate, frightening place, devoid of alternatives and hope. Traumatic experiences have the power to anchor the individual in a cramped place from which all too often the only horizon seen is the limits created by one's defenses. If trauma can be considered the opposite of empowerment (Levine, 2010), the goal of any effective intervention is to support the individual in moving out of a defensive state by creating a context that makes this first step feel solid and safe enough.

There is no single path to recovery from trauma. An effective intervention in crisis contexts is one that avoids forcing entry into the castle and instead offers a multitude of sources and alternatives for connection, involvement, acquisition, and strengthening of capabilities, elaboration of past experiences, and definition of future paths. The challenges are many, including the need to make the terrain as safe and rich in possibilities as possible while keeping in mind that what is inviting and stimulating for one person, may not be so for the other or may not even be suitable for a specific context.

All the considerations made lead us to a great truth: there is no intervention more effective than the one that respects the times and spaces of one's interlocutors, without giving in to external pressures but valuing the wisdom of those who are the only ones who can truly regain possession of their present and build their future.

## REFERENCES

Bettelheim, B. (1987). The importance of play. *The Atlantic, 259*(3). https://www.theatlantic.com/magazine/archive/1987/03/the-importance-of-play/305129/

Cassina, I. (2023). Recovering lost play time. Principles and intervention modalities to address the psychosocial wellbeing of asylum seekers and refugee children. In I. Cassina, C. Mochi, & K. Stagnitti (Eds.), *Play therapy and expressive arts in a complex and dynamic world: Opportunities and challenges inside and outside the playroom* (pp. 50–68). Routledge.

Cassina, I., & Mochi, C. (2023). Applying the therapeutic power of play and expressive arts in contemporary crisis work. A process-oriented approach. In I. Cassina, C. Mochi, & K. Stagnitti (Eds.), *Play therapy and expressive arts in a complex and dynamic world: Opportunities and challenges inside and outside the playroom* (pp. 6–27). Routledge.

Ginsburg, K. R. (2007). The importance of play in promoting healthy child development and maintaining strong parent-child bonds. *Pediatrics, 119*(1), 182–191.

Halprin, D. (1999). Living artfully. Movement as an integrative process. In S. K. Levine & E. G. Levine (Eds.), *Foundations of expressive arts therapy theoretical and clinical perspectives* (pp. 133–149). Jessica Kingsley Publishers.

van der Kolk, B. (2014). *The body keeps the score: Brain, mind, and body in the healing of trauma*. Penguin Books.

Levine, P. A. (2010). *In an unspoken voice: How the body releases trauma and restores goodness*. North Atlantic Books.

Levine, S. K. (2019). *Philosophy of expressive arts therapy: Poiesis and the therapeutic imagination*. Jessica Kingsley Publishers.

MacFarlane, A. C. (1987). Posttraumatic phenomenon in a longitudinal study of children following natural disaster. *Journal of the American Academy of Child and Adolescent Psychiatry, 26*(5), 764–769.

Malchiodi, C. A. (2020). *Trauma and expressive arts therapy: Brain, body, and imagination in the healing process*. The Guilford Press.

Masten, A. S., & Cicchetti, D. (2010). Developmental cascades [Editorial]. *Development and Psychopathology, 22*(3), 491–495. https://doi.org/10.1017/S0954579410000222.

Masten, A. S., & Narayan, A. J. (2011). Child development in the context of disaster, war, and terrorism: Pathways of risk and resilience. *Annual Review of Psychology,63*(1),227–257.https://www.annualreviews.org/doi/10.1146/annurev-psych-120710-100356

Mochi, C. (2022). *Beyond the clouds: An autoethnographic research exploring the good practice in crisis settings*. Loving Healing Press.

Mochi, C., & Cassina, I. (2024). Reclaiming a feeling of safety in natural disasters: Preparatory and advanced interventions using play and play therapy. In P. Goodyear-Brown & L. Yasenik (Eds.), *Polyvagal power in the playroom*. Routledge.

Mochi, C., & Stagnitti, K. (2023). Learn to play therapy in high-risk countries. The example of Nigeria. In I. Cassina, C. Mochi, & K. Stagnitti (Eds.), *Play therapy and expressive arts in a complex and dynamic world: Opportunities and challenges inside and outside the playroom* (pp. 96–119). Routledge.

Perry, B. D. (2007). Stress, trauma and post-traumatic stress disorders in children. *The Child Trauma Academy, 17*, 42–57.

Perry, B. D., Pollard, R. A., Blakley, T. L., Baker, W. L., & Vigilante, D. (1995). Childhood trauma, the neurobiology of adaptation, and "use-dependent" development of the brain: How "states" become "traits". *Infant Mental Health Journal, 16*(4), 271–291.

Porges, S. W. (2015). Making the world safe for our children: Downregulating defence and up-regulating social engagement to 'optimise' the human experience. *Children Australia, 40*(02), 114–123.

Porges, S. W. (2017). *The pocket guide to the polyvagal theory: The transformative power of feeling safe*. Norton & Company.

Porges, S. W. (2021). *Polyvagal safety: Attachment, communication, self-regulation*. (IPNB). Norton & Company.

Sameroff, A. J., Seifer, R., Barocas, R., Zax, M., & Greenspan, S. (1987). Intelligence quotient scores of 4-year-old children: Social-environmental risk factors. *Pediatrics, 79*(3), 343–350.

Schaefer, C. E., & Drewes, A. A. (2014). *The therapeutic powers of play: 20 core agents of change* ((2nd ed.). ed.). Wiley.

Schore, A. N. (2019). *The development of the unconscious mind*. Norton & Company.

Shore, R. (1997). *Rethinking the brain*. Families and Work Institute.

VanFleet, R., Sywulak, A. E., & Sniscak, C. C. (Eds.) (2010). *Child-centered play therapy*. The Guilford Press.

Yehuda, R., Teicher, M. H., Seckl, J., Grossman, R. A., Morris, A., & Bierer, L. M. (2007). Parental posttraumatic stress disorder as a vulnerability factor for low cortisol trait in offspring of Holocaust survivors. *Archives of General Psychiatry, 64*(9), 1040–1048.

## CHAPTER FIFTEEN

# Inoculation, Protection, and Processing: The Powers of Video Game Use with Trauma

JESSICA STONE

As discussed in numerous ways throughout this text, trauma weaves a poisonous web for individuals, families, and societies. These singular or serried events pose a threat to a person's physical and/or psychological well-being. As a society, we have the important tasks of preventing, protecting against, and processing traumas, depending on our roles and responsibilities. Mental health practitioners have a particularly vital role in this dynamic. We can ask ourselves, "In what ways can I best assist my clients before, during, and after traumatic events?"

The current digital technology era includes a host of software, hardware, and platforms, which provide extensive and complex experiences for the participant. As described by Ceranoglu (2010), Stone (2019, 2020, 2022, 2023), and Granic et al. (2014), there are a plethora of benefits to the inclusion of video games in the mental health trauma treatment process. The more we understand what is happening for the individual regarding the traumatic experience(s), the more we can identify and connect these concepts with the components of digital play. This chapter serves to build the bridge and provide the known underpinnings to date of both the impact of trauma on the being, and the therapeutic use of video games within the inoculation, protection, and processing phases of mental health treatment. Beginning with the brain, mind, and body fundamentals, as well as learning and memory consolidation processes, the impacts of primary and secondary trauma will be explored for both the individual and the collective through the identification of gameplay components and effects.

## THE BRAIN, THE MIND, AND THE BODY

The presentation of video game therapy, a component of Digital Play Therapy™, as a mental health treatment modality for primary (a direct and immediate exposure to a distressing event or experience) and secondary trauma (the indirect exposure to trauma experienced by others) experiences is grounded in components of the bodily processes and video game play (Stone, 2019, 2020, 2021, 2022, 2023). A brief orientation to the concepts allows the connective bridge between each to be established.

In recognizing the brain–mind–body connection, Stone states that "even if we think we are speaking to and with one portion of the brain, we are actually activating millions of neurons throughout the brain, mind, and body" (2023, p. 51). The recognition of the inherent interconnectedness, and therefore both the vulnerability and power, of the impact of the experiences one has on the holistic being informs *everything* we do as humans.

Damasio describes that there is an interplay between the brain, mind, and body:

1. The human brain and the rest of the body constitute an indissociable organism, integrated by means of mutually interactive biochemical and neural regulatory circuits (including endocrine, immune, and autonomic neural components).
2. The organism interacts with the environment as an ensemble: the interaction is neither of the body alone or the brain alone.
3. The physiological operations that we call mind are derived from the structural and functional ensemble rather than from the brain alone: mental phenomena can be fully understood only in the context of an organism interacting in an environment. (2005, pp. xx–xxi)

## THE BRAIN

Johns Hopkins Medicine defines the brain as "a complex organ that controls thought, memory, emotion, touch, motor skills, vision, breathing, temperature, hunger and every process that regulates our body." (2023, para. 1). The brain is the organizing power center of our being; the hub of body's abilities to receive, perceive, and produce. This three-pound organ is the "intelligence, interpreter of the senses, initiator of body movement, and controller of behavior" for the body (NIH, 2022, para. 1). Originally conceptualized as a collection of distinct components, the brain is now known as an "extensively distributed set of neurons we call the 'nervous system' and its many components that are interwoven with the body as a whole" (Siegel, 2012, p. xxi).

*For our current purpose, the key importance of our understanding of the brain is the recognition of the interconnectedness to everything in the being, and therefore, how traumatic experiences can impact the entirety of being in a burst of electrical impulses.*

## THE MIND

An abstract and seldomly agreed upon concept, the mind has numerous definitions. Definitions of the mind from anthropologists ("what is shared across the generations") to neuroscientists ("the mind is simply the activity of the brain") to psychologists ("the mind is composed of thoughts and feelings and includes our consciousness and the subjective nature of our internal lives as well as the output of the mind, which are our behaviors.") indicate the difficulty in defining what the conceptualization of the mind actually is (Siegel, 2012, p. xxi; Stone, 2023).

Despite these difficulties, holding space for the concept of the mind as a component of consciousness distinguishes it from the mechanics of electricity and function. "The mind is process and action (or the conscious outcome of process and action), the brain is the mechanism in which that action occurs. While the brain can exist without the mind, the converse is certainly not true." (Uttal, 1987, p. 672).

*The inclusion of the mind in the discussion of the inoculation, protection, and processing of trauma speaks to the consciousness of the experiences and includes ties directly to the brain and body.*

## THE BODY

For the purposes of this chapter, the discussion regarding the body will focus on interoception. In 1906, Sherrington introduced the concept of interoception in his book, *Integrative Action of the Nervous System* (1947). Stemming from the medicalized definitions of that era, Sherrington's definition referred to the physiological manifestations, internal perceptions, and awareness of stimuli recognized and interpreted by the body.

*The importance of the recognition of bodily manifestations of internal states is key to the conceptualizations of the impacts of trauma.*

A more current definition provided by Chen et al., (2021), posits that interoception is "the representation of an organism's internal states, and includes the processes by which it senses, interprets, integrates, and regulates signals from within itself." (para. 1). Sensations that manifest physically translate into emotional sensations through the interplay between the autonomic nervous system (ANS) and the central nervous system (CNS) (Candia-Rivera et al., 2022; Stone, 2023). The communication between the ANS and the CNS through interoceptive neural circuits contributes to decision-making, the creation of feelings, and emotional experiences (Azzalini et al., 2021; Candia-Rivera et al., 2022; Chen et al., 2021; Fujimoto et al., 2021; Stone, 2023).

*Interoception allows for the awareness and mindfulness of the impacts of traumatic stimuli and experiences on the brain, mind, and body and leads to the connection of concepts within video game play.*

The mind, brain, and body allow for interconnectedness, consciousness, awareness, and mindfulness in all we do. When we engage in an experience, we are activating these complex systems in preparation for, and in reaction to, a variety of stimuli. A brief peek into the processes of cognition, learning, and engagement will help us to understand what happens when the stimuli "enters the body" (through any of the senses), how do we process it, and how might that be impacted in positive and negative ways?

## COGNITION, LEARNING, AND ENGAGEMENT

To learn we must employ processes of cognition. Neisser (1967) referred to cognition as "all the processes by which the sensory input is transformed, reduced, elaborated, stored, recovered, and used." He continues with "such terms as sensation, perception, imagery, retention, recall, problem-solving, and thinking, among many others, refer to hypothetical stages or aspects of cognition." (p. 4). Cognition allows us to process information for organization, learning, and engagement.

How we learn and engage impacts the connections of neural networks and the organization of information within the brain. Neural nets, or networks, transmit information by connecting based on the determined importance and relevance of the information (weight of the signal) (Bingham & Miikkulainen, 2022). Imagine the neural dendrites reaching out and grabbing like-"minded" neurons and holding on tight because they have similarities; they have strength in numbers. In response to trauma, this impacts the understanding and organization of the stimuli, which in turn impacts brain–mind–body triggers. Traumatic triggers can affect a person's day-to-day living on both conscious and unconscious levels.

To engage in something is to "take part in something" (Cambridge Dictionary, 2023, para. 1). When we are engaged in something, these networks within the brain–mind–body activate for participation. This participation can be for the positive (conversation, relationships, activities, etc.) or the negative (survival, preservation, risk-mitigation, etc.). When people are engaged, alert, and thinking (cognition), we can create a state-dependent environment, which can impact the treatment of those who have experienced trauma. Perceived environments and experiences can trigger state-dependent experiences, which can become a central part of trauma treatment.

When trauma occurs, the mind, brain, and body activate in a flurry of determinations of safety, action, reaction, strategy, and more. In the interest of safety, engagement, cognitions, and neural network connections can and will be made between the trauma and past and current experiences, leaving space for the connections to future ones as well. Part of the trauma therapy process is to identify these connections and (a) determine if they are connected properly (maybe the connection was made in haste due to safety concerns?) and (b) how might they be connected/organized differently to serve the person more accurately?

Understanding learning serves three primary functions in our understanding of trauma impacts: (a) inoculation, or the experiences and information utilized for preparation and anticipation of trauma, (b) protection, the organization and processing of the trauma(s) and the minimization of the impacts, and (c) process, or the expression, creation, and catharsis to reorganize the neural networks and possibly the transition of traumas from short-term to long-term memory in a healthier, more adaptive manner.

*Each of these concepts contributes to the bridge between the internal and external experiences of the client and the modality of utilizing video games in therapy. Through the understanding of the ways trauma is perceived, organized, stored, and experienced, we can better pair therapeutic interventions, which allow the client to heal.*

## VIDEO GAMES IN TRAUMA THERAPY

Digital tools used in therapy can offer millions of possibilities in environment, creation, interaction, identification, representation, and so on. Video games in trauma therapy can capitalize on that which the client and/or clinician identify as therapeutically relevant. Traditional therapeutic tools have much less available flexibility. Both the client and the clinician, or together as a team, can work to identify the components of the interaction that will elicit change in the brain–mind–body, cognition, learning, and engagement processes. Colors, sounds, and visuals can be chosen and even created; types of roles can be identified, tried, and explored; interactions can be sought out, avoided, and explored. These components can be part of an abreactive, cathartic, or exploratory process, which advances the treatment plan, and the client's functioning forward in an organic, familiar, controlled, and intentional way.

## RESEARCH

Many clinicians will be surprised to learn of the impressive body of research involving the use of video games in therapy. To list only a few, studies that include concepts pertinent to this topic include those that explore cognitive enhancement, positive emotions, and sensorimotor systems (Franceschini et al., 2022; Hastings, 2022), strength and resilience (Kelly, 2020), social and emotional health, (McMahan, 2022), trauma-informed virtual reality (Stone, 2021), and the development of a "cognitive vaccine" against traumatic flashbacks (Holmes et al., 2010, p. 2; Iyadurai et al., 2018).

Of particular interest to this chapter is the work by Holmes et al. (2010) and Iyadurai et al. (2018). These two studies focus on the use of the video game Tetris, a visuospatial task game created in 1984 by Alexey Pajitnov (Holmes et al., 2010; Tetris, 2023). These researchers set out to find "evidence-based methods to prevent the build-up of symptoms" of post-traumatic stress disorder (PTSD) because "we lack early interventions to treat people in the aftermath of trauma exposure" (Holmes et al., 2010, p. 1).

In the first experiment of the Holmes et al. study, they presented 66 non-clinical subjects with a traumatic film followed by a 30-minute break, and neutral static slides from the film. Subjects were then randomly assigned to one of three groups: Tetris, no task, or a computerized Pub Quiz game for 10 minutes. The subjects "had significantly fewer intrusions whilst playing Tetris compared to the no-task condition with no comparable difference between the Pub Quiz game and no-task condition" (p. 2). After leaving, the subjects were asked to keep a structured diary to record their flashbacks or "involuntary visual mental images" of the trauma film for the next week (p. 2). The Tetris group reported, "significantly fewer flashbacks over the week than both the no task (d = .70) and Pub Quiz (d = 1.21) conditions" (p. 2). Interestingly, the group that played the Pub Quiz game had a significant increase in flashbacks over the week compared to the no-task group.

For the second experiment of the first Holmes et al. study (2010), 75 non-clinical participants watched the same film and then left the facility for 4 hours to do as they pleased. Upon return, they were assigned to the groups as delineated above, including the stimulus reminder, and they were asked to keep a diary of flashbacks for a week. Again, the Tetris group experienced significantly fewer flashbacks compared to the other groups. These second experiment findings show that even with a delay in the Tetris gameplay, the group reported significantly fewer flashbacks. Again, the group that played the Pub Quiz game had a significant increase in flashbacks over the week compared to the no-task group. The authors posit that "verbal/conceptual interference may worsen flashbacks in the consolidation phase" of memory (Holmes et al., 2010, p. 6).

Let us digest that for a moment. These two experiments found that people who were exposed to traumatic material played a simple visuospatial task video game, Tetris, up to 4 full hours after exposure and reported *significantly fewer flashbacks for a week* after the experiment. The Pub Quiz, a verbal/conceptual task, generated significantly more flashbacks. Why is this? What value does the visuospatial computer-generated task bring that serves as an inoculation against a key element of PTSD? Because cognitive science studies show that cognitive, visuospatial tasks compete for brain–mind–body resources with visual images—the visuospatial task occupies space, energy, and *neural net weight* that would otherwise be dedicated to the traumatic visual images and diverting them from forming as many or as substantial neural networks as someone who had not played the game. This reduces the systems that would have produced flashbacks and triggers.

The second study by Iyadurai et al. (2018) sought to re-test the Holmes et al. study and find a "low-intensity psychiatric intervention that could prevent debilitating memories following trauma" (p. 1). This study took place in an emergency department with people who had experienced the real-life trauma of a motor vehicle accident. Building off of memory consolidation theory (McGaugh, 1966, 2000) and the historic, yet still valid perseveration–consolidation hypothesis of memory (Müller & Pilzecker, 1900), it is believed that "memory of newly learned information was disrupted by the learning of other information shortly after the original learning and suggested that processes underlying new memories initially persist in a fragile state and consolidate over time" (McGaugh, 2000, p. 248).

Given that Holmes et al. (2010) found that engaging in visuospatial tasks assisted with a reduction in flashbacks, Iyudurai et al. set out to test their hypothesis that cognitive tasks that are high in visuospatial demands during the time of "trauma memory consolidation may reduce the occurrence of subsequent intrusive visual memories of trauma" (2018, p. 675). The study included 71 patients who presented to the emergency department in Oxford, UK, and participated within 6 hours of their accident. The participants were split into 2 groups, one of which was a control group and the other recalled the trauma briefly and then played Tetris for 10 uninterrupted minutes, followed by an outcome assessment at the 1 week and 1 month[1] anniversary of the accident. The study found a *62% reduction* in the number of intrusive memories when compared to the control group at the 1-week assessment. Those who did report intrusive memories reported that they diminished more quickly than the control group (Iyadarai et al., 2018).

---

[1] The findings at the 1-month mark were considered negligible for each group and better determined through a larger sample size in future studies.

With concerns about historical approaches to trauma treatment, such as Critical Incident Stress Debriefing (U.S. Department of Veterans Affairs, 2022) and medications that have drawbacks, an alternative that provides symptom reduction is important to find (Holmes et al., 2010). These two studies have shown reliability over time and with different levels of experience and stimuli that cognitive visuospatial tasks provided through an engaging video game medium have a significant impact on intrusive memories and flashbacks of a traumatic event.

## INOCULATION, PROTECTION, AND PROCESSING

Given what we have explored about the brain–mind–body, learning, cognition, engagement, and memory consolidation, along with the power of a cognitive visuospatial video game as one example of a therapeutic video game intervention, we can explore forms of therapeutic application. We will look to ways of inoculation (the experiences and information utilized for preparation and anticipation of trauma), protection (the organization and processing of the trauma[s] and the minimization of the impacts), and process (the expression, creation, catharsis, etc., of working through trauma).

## COMPONENTS WITHIN THE GAMEPLAY PROCESS

Within this gameplay process, the user can work toward any number of therapeutic goals and skills. A common guidance when people are feeling hopeless, helpless, or stuck is to help them "identify the helpers." This may be worded differently for different age groups, but the concept is the same—who can be of help in a situation; what constitutes the person's support system; how can a person who has been impacted by trauma(s) identify the need for help, identify what or who could be helpful, seek out the help, and accept the help? One way this could manifest in a video game is through the assistance of others within the game, whether that be an in-game non-player character (NPC; a character in the game, which does not have a human playing the character), another human character, a peer or friend, a YouTube video, or a website.

Perspective is another important component of trauma treatment. Sometimes we can get lost in a particular aspect or view and there is power in looking at the dynamic from a different angle. At times, it is important to look at the big picture, the overall umbrella of a situation. At other times, exploration at the microcosm level is the most powerful; those of the smallest detail. This can be as simple as a shift in vantage point by discussing a gameplay scenario as the view is rotated, zoomed in, or zoomed out. It can be a more complex process with the client embodying different characters or roles. The possibilities are endless.

The identification and exploration of needs can lead to problem-solving and coping skill experiences and conversations. The trial-and-error possibilities within the play and the control to begin, stop, and change the engagement within the play allow the client to be the master of their domain. As one example, frustration can certainly arise within the play, but it is less the existence of the frustration, and more the self-regulation and management of the frustration (frustration tolerance), which can be addressed in these situations.

Identifying goals and the necessary tasks and/or steps to achieve them is another experience available in video gameplay. Exploring the map, the stated quests, and the desired achievement(s) are all easily attainable features within video games. Critically thinking through the tasks, the pros and cons, the dangers, and the safeties allows the user to identify steps to take and ways to keep one's self safe. At times, people who have experienced trauma(s) have lost (or may have never established) their own sense of personal agency (sense of control and autonomy). Video gameplay can allow for the exploration and practice toward these important competencies.

Video gameplay within therapeutic sessions also allows for opportunities to learn about ways to keep one's self safe, both emotionally and physically. With a sense of "other," or separateness possible in some games (lower levels of immersion and embodiment), the player can evaluate their own characters as well as any others in the game. At other times, the increased immersion and embodiment, also known as ownership, can lead to personal insights and self-evaluations. Since the gameplay can be anywhere on the spectrum from a 2-dimensional (2D) interactive experience (i.e., a computer or console game) to a 3-dimensional (3D) experience (i.e., virtual, augmented, or mixed reality), the clinician can provide the environment that matches the needs.

## DIFFERENT PHASES FOR DIFFERENT NEEDS: APPLYING THE VIDEO GAME COMPONENTS

### INOCULATION

An inoculation is a vaccine; an introduction of material formulated to expose the body to something that will trigger a protective response in hopes of fighting off a threat. A therapeutic video game intervention geared toward trauma inoculation will allow the user opportunities for practice, trial and error, strategy, cause and effect, micro- and macro- perspectives of a situation, and multi-sequential tasks. The user is exposed to doses of stressful situations with the ability to learn how to manage them. This can be in anticipation of a particular situation or dynamic, or in general for day-to-day life. Providing a scaffold for the brain–mind–body and a pre-organized system for cognition and memory consolidation can assist when trauma occurs.

*An example of when an inoculation could be used would be when there is an anticipated loss.*

## Protection

The protection process can be utilized at any time, and for our purposes, is thought of as a mid-experience component of trauma treatment. If the inoculation process had been in place, recalling the experiences and skills within those interactions would be beneficial. In this treatment stage, it is important for the clinician to connect, join, and hold the space for the experience as it is happening. It is common for an array of emotional and behavioral expressions to occur, and the variety of available video games, from active to creative—passive to immersive, can allow outlets for each. Keeping oneself safe and learning to both express and regulate through this phase allows for stability, thereby acting as protection for the self. This is when the neural networks are working to connect, and visuospatial tasks such as the use of Tetris can assist in keeping the strength of those painful networks from forming.

*An example of when protection could be used would be during current happenings of a loss.*

## Processing

A goal to process the aftermath or consequences of trauma may be the most common within mental health treatment. Creating and providing safe, organic environments for catharsis, abreaction, expression, or soothing after one has experienced the trauma(s) allows the client to become more in tune with their internal responses. Video gameplay environments allow for the expression of any experience, including the "ugly" portions we rarely want anyone to see. We can go into an environment (2D or 3D) and destroy it and yell, scream, and cry, or organize it to make sense of it all, or anywhere in between. Through these experiences, we can form new neural network pairings, which allow space for healing and shifts from hopelessness and helplessness to strength and mastery.

*An example of when processing could be used would be during the aftermath of a loss.*

## CASE EXAMPLES

Three mini-case examples will be presented here to briefly illustrate each of the three stages of trauma care discussed in this chapter. Each example highlights the use of Digital Play Therapy.

## INOCULATION

Sadie was a 16-year-old who presented to treatment with fears that her parents were heading toward a divorce. Even though they had not spoken with her about it, she was attending to their behaviors and level of fighting and found herself stressed about the possibility. With a focus on her own locus of control, the clinician and Sadie explored ways she could regulate herself when she felt these stressors, and how she might look at her parent's situation from different perspectives.

To create an environment for these explorations, Tilt Brush in virtual reality was the chosen medium. Tilt Brush is a program that allows the user to draw and create 3D art in many colors and styles. For Sadie, it was a way to create a safe space for herself, with sounds happening with each brushstroke, and the control of the appearance, size, and color of her creations. Since the creation was 3D, she was able to go inside her creation and embellish it in ways that were meaningful to her.

Exploring the situation for herself had importance, as well as imagining what her parent's perspectives might be. She created representations of her parents in Tilt Brush and included thought bubbles for each with what they might be thinking and feeling. She rotated her own body around each of them to literally have a different view while she drew, wrote, and spoke about each aspect. She felt a tremendous amount of relief and created ways to self-soothe and organize incoming information from her parents, if she needed to in the future.

## PROTECTION

Christopher was a 33-year-old client who was in the midst of experiencing the death of his father. His goals included creating a space to hold his many emotions and protect him from catastrophizing and generalizing globally about the meaninglessness of life, which he had done before in less personal situations.

Zelda, Breath of the Wild, is an adventure game where the main character, Link, must accept many challenges, defeat the ultimate evil, restore peace, and save the kingdom of Hyrule. For Christopher, this environment provided a number of elements he needed at this time; he was able to run in fields and look off enormous cliffs; he shrieked while he fought off trolls and other enemies. He would exclaim, breathe, and yell while playing the game. He teared up a bit when he tamed a horse and rode it wildly through the land as he shared that he and his father used to ride horses together when he was a child. At one point, he flung himself (Link, the character he was playing) off the cliff to his death and stated that he would never do that in real life, but it felt good to do that in the game. He quickly reset his character and moved on to a different task.

Having the space to express the many emotions he was having, along with acting out in ways he would not in his day-to-day life allowed the weight of his emotions to lessen. Standing in the fields and riding the horse reminded him of the good times and the beauty of life, which decreased his tendency to catastrophize and focus on the parts of his relationship with his father that he would miss. He was able to gain a new perspective about the pending loss of his father.

## Processing

Marly, a sullen and withdrawn 9-year-old, presented for treatment with her father. Her mother had recently died in a car accident and she and her father were both experiencing raw and painful impacts of their loss. It was discovered through the intake that Marly had been in the car during the accident, sustained her own injuries, and watched as the responders attempted to save her mother.

During the initial meetings, it was discovered that Marly enjoyed playing Animal Crossing: New Horizons (ACNH), a multiplayer game on the Nintendo Switch. Each player has an island, animal neighbors, a home to decorate, and items to gather and craft. Players can visit each other's islands and explore together. She was willing to play the game and visit the clinician's island. She was not initially ready to share her own.

After exploring the clinician's island, fishing and swimming together, wandering around the museum and coffee shop, and chatting with the island residents, Marly decided it was time to allow the clinician to visit her island. Her island was primarily orderly with flowers adorning the buildings and pathways. Her house was up on a hill, overlooking the water. Below the house, though, was a very chaotic, weed-filled, neglected area. She stated she didn't like that spot and did not know what to do with it.

Based on numerous accounts during COVID-19 (the game launched at the beginning of the pandemic), ACNH has been frequently used as a vehicle to honor and grieve for those who have died (Carpenter, 2020; DaRienzo, 2020; Medina, 2020). The clinicians shared a few of the ways people were honoring those they had lost on their islands, and Marly decided she wanted to use the neglected area in this way. She spent time carefully creating and populating the area as a love and honor to her mother. The clinician and Marly visited the area during each session and placed flowers together. She was able to share memories and an array of emotions she was experiencing. It was incredibly powerful and moving to bear witness to her grief and healing.

## THE FUTURE

The future of the use of digital tools, and specifically video games, in trauma work is ever-expanding and ripe for application. As with any therapeutic intervention, it is imperative that the clinician attend to the 5Cs: Comfort, Competence, Culture, Congruence, and Capability (Stone, 2022), which include and address important ethical issues within the work. It is important that we are open to the inclusion and value of video games, and the powers within, to provide the experiences necessary within the brain–mind–body.

Psychology as a field will benefit from each of us contributing to the future development of the games and spaces, the guidelines and the standards, and the infusion of important psychological concepts into the programs. The multilayered, multidimensional experiences within the gameplay speak to the human condition, the past, present, and the future of goals and needs, the learnings and understandings, and the emotions and reactions. The possibilities really are endless.

## CONCLUSION

The exploration of the process with which a person experiences trauma inside their brain–mind–body provides a structure within which we can understand further how video games can meet important needs. Digital technology software, hardware, and platforms provide extensive and complex experiences for the participant, which address the needs of a client. The more we understand what is happening for the individual regarding the traumatic experience(s), the more we can identify and connect these concepts with the components of the digital play.

Within this chapter, we have created a bridge between the internal processes of trauma in the brain–mind–body and the therapeutic use of video games to inoculate, protect, and process one's experience. Armed with the power of these digital tools, clinicians can expand their repertoire of offerings to meet their clients' needs at a deeper and more intimate level. Providing the environment and experiences that maximize healing promotes healing in the most difficult of times.

## REFERENCES

Azzalini, D., Buot, A., Palminteri, S., & Tallon-Baudry, C. (2021). Responses to heartbeats in ventromedial prefrontal cortex contribute to subjective preference-based decisions. *Journal of Neuroscience, 41*(23), 5102–5114.

Bingham, G., & Miikkulainen, R. (2022). *AutoInit: Analytic signal-preserving weight initialization for neural networks.* Association for the Advancement of Artificial Intelligence. https://arxiv.org/pdf/2109.08958.pdf

Cambridge Dictionary (2023). *Engage in something.* https://dictionary.cambridge.org/dictionary/english/engage-in

Candia-Rivera, D., Catrambone, V., Thayer, J. F., Gentili, C., & Valenza, G. (2022). Cardiac sympathetic-vagal activity initiates a functional brain-body response to emotional arousal. *PNAS, 119*(21). https://www.pnas.org/doi/10.1073/pnas.2119599119

Carpenter, N. (2020). *Animal crossing players are building in-game memorials: 'It's kind of like she's living on in the game': Technology has influenced how we grieve. Polygon.* https://www.polygon.com/2020/7/1/21309893/animal-crossing-new-horizons-memorials-nintendo-grief

Ceranoglu, T. A. (2010). Video games in psychotherapy. *Review of General Psychology, APA, 14*(2), 141–146.

Chen, W. G., Schloesser, D., Arensdorf, A. M., Simmons, J. M., Cui, C., Valentino, R., Gnadt, J. W., Nielsen, L., St. Hillare-Clarke, C., Spruance, V., Horowitzz, T. S., Vallejo, Y. F., & Langecin, H. M. (2021). The emerging science of interoception: Sensing, integrating, interpreting, and regulating signals from within the self. *Trends Neurocience, 44*(1), 3–16. https://doi.org/10.1016/j.tins.2020.10.007

Damasio, A. (2005). *Descartes' error: Emotion, reason, and the human brain.* Penguin.

DaRienzo, G. (2020). *Exploring grief in animal crossing: New Horizons.* The Order of the Good Death. https://www.orderofthegooddeath.com/article/exploring-grief-in-animal-crossing-new-horizons/

Franceschini, S., Bertoni, S., Lulli, M., Pievani, T., & Facoetti, A. (2022). Short-term effects of video-games on cognitive enhancement: The role of positive emotions. *Journal of Cognitive Enhancement, 6,* 29–46.

Fujimoto, A., Murray, E. A., & Rudebeck, P. H. (2021). *Interaction between decision-making and interoceptive representations of bodily arousal in frontal cortex. NIH.* https://www.ncbi.nlm.nih.gov/pmc/articles/PMC8536360/pdf/pnas.202014781.pdf

Granic, I., Lobel, A., & Engels, R. (2014). The benefits of gaming. *American Psychologist, 69*(1), 66–78.

Hastings, C. (2022, October 11). *Video games to improve cognition in older adults.* https://www.medgadget.com/2022/10/video-games-to-improve-cognition-in-older-adults.html?fbclid=IwAR3I4c6Xxb-CCMQNZD0skgmd3EIrevhnpXhOxrC6M4nOX9DmHDA2INbIo_M

Holmes, E. A., James, E. L., Kilford, E. J., & Deeprose, C. (2010). Key steps in developing a cognitive vaccine against traumatic flashbacks: Visuospatial Tetris versus verbal Pub Quiz. *PLoS One, 5*(11), 1–9.

Iyadurai, L., Blackwell, S. E., Meiser-Stedman, R., Watson, P. C., Bonsall, M. B., Geddes, J. R., Nobre, A. C., & Holmes, E. A. (2018). Preventing intrusive memories after trauma via a brief intervention involving Tetris computer game play in the emergency department: A proof-of-concept randomized controlled trial. *Molecular Psychiatry, 23,* 674–682.

Johns Hopkins Medicine (2023). *Brain anatomy and how the brain works.* Hopkins Medicine.https://www.hopkinsmedicine.org/health/conditions-and-diseases/anatomy-of-the-brain

Kelly, R. (2020). Positive psychology and gaming: Strength and resilience. In R. Kowert's (Ed.), *Video games and well-being: Press start* (pp. 77–96). Palgrave MacMillon.

McGaugh, J. L. (1966). Time-dependent processes in memory storage. *Science, 153,* 1351–1358.

McGaugh, J. L. (2000). Memory—A century of consolidation. *Science, 287,* 248–251.

McMahan, L. (2022, November 23). *Video games support young patients' social, emotional health.*https://news.ohsu.edu/2022/11/23/video-games-support-young-patients-social-emotional-health?fbclid=IwAR3cDj_vtWUxstbv4Ib5a2c49LHHyYpQ3MLoK07vD943lJeA6LqScbxdZt8

Medina, J. (2020). *Using animal crossing for the grieving process. Guidance Teletherapy.* https://www.guidancett.com/blog/using-animal-crossing-for-the-grieving-process-2021

Müller, G. E., & Pilzecker, A. (1900). Experimentelle Beitrage zur Lehre vom Gedachtniss [Experimental contributions to the theory of memory]. *A. Psychol, 1,* 1–288. https://ia800407.us.archive.org/25/items/b28111916/b28111916.pdf

Neisser, E. (1967). *Cognitive psychology.* Appleton-Century-Crofts.

NIH (2022). *Brain basics: Know your brain. National Institute of Neurological Disorders and Stroke.* https://www.ninds.nih.gov/health-information/patient-caregiver-education/brain-basics-know-your-brain

Sherrington, C. S. (1947). *Integrative action of the nervous system.* Cambridge. (Original work published 1906).

Siegel, D. J. (2012). *Pocket guide to interpersonal biology: An integrative handbook of the mind.* Norton.

Stone, J. (2019). Digital games. In J. Stone & C. E. Schaefer (Eds.), *Game play* (3rd ed., pp. 99–115). Wiley.

Stone, J. (2020). *Digital play therapy: A clinician's guide to comfort and competence* (1st ed.). Routledge.

Stone, J. (2021, fall/winter). Trauma-informed virtual reality play. *Playground Magazine,* 13–16.

Stone, J. (2022). *Digital play therapy: A clinician's guide to comfort and competence* (2nd ed.). Routledge.

Stone, J. (2023). *Technology in mental health: Foundations of clinical use.* Routledge.

Tetris (2023). *Corporate bios.* https://tetris.com/bios

U.S. Department of Veterans Affairs (2022). *PTSD: National center for PTSD.* https://www.ptsd.va.gov/professional/treat/type/debrief_after_disasters.asp

Uttal, W. R. (1987). Mind, the psychobiology of. In G. Adelman (Ed.), *Encyclopedia of neuroscience* (Vol. II, pp. 672–674). Birkhäuser.

## CHAPTER SIXTEEN

# Utilizing Tabletop Roleplaying Games in Treating Trauma and Post-Traumatic Stress Disorder

BRIAN QUINONES and SHELBY SOMERS

## TRAUMA AND PTSD

### TRAUMA

Over the past decade, the understanding and treatment of trauma have grown significantly. It is estimated that 16% of children and young people will be exposed to traumatic events, leading to post-traumatic stress disorder (PTSD) (Mavranezouli et al., 2020a). Additionally, PTSD is estimated to impact nearly eight million adults in the United States alone (Butler et al., 2020). In more recent years, we have found that previous understandings of what a traumatic event consists of and how that trauma impacts the individual and society have evolved. Existing research (Evans, 2020; Humble et al., 2019) demonstrates the negative impact traumatic events have on individuals and the long-lasting adverse effects on the individual's physical, social, emotional, mental, spiritual well-being, and development. Trauma increases the risk of other health-related concerns if left untreated. As a result, there is a need to explore different approaches to address trauma and the comorbid symptoms.

When looking to address and treat trauma, it is important to explore the needs of the individual. Often, individuals who have experienced a traumatic event or have been diagnosed with PTSD experience a sense of isolation and

*Trauma Impacts: The Repercussions of Individual and Collective Trauma*, First Edition.
Edited by Jessica Stone, Robert J. Grant, and Clair Mellenthin.
© 2024 John Wiley & Sons, Inc. Published 2024 by John Wiley & Sons, Inc.

loneliness (Sloan et al., 2012). It can be difficult to trust, connect, and return to a previous sense of safety. It is because of these challenges that individuals often present with a need for connection. While this certainly begins as part of the therapeutic process in individual sessions, group psychotherapy and support can also work to develop connections while also giving space for catharsis and processing. Since every individual is different and experiences trauma in different ways, there is an increased need to explore other approaches to building connection, resilience, and allowing for catharsis.

Tabletop Roleplaying games (TTRPGs) are a shared storytelling experience where actions, settings, and characters are described verbally. While there are various game mechanics that can lead to different player experiences, generally, dice or cards are involved to determine if actions are successful. TTRPGs have a wide variety of themes and forms of roleplaying. For example, while typically TTRPGs have a game master (GM) who is the predominant narrator of the story for players, there are also TTRPGs that have a shared GM or no GM at all. This means that the players work together to tell a collaborative story through their roleplay. There is also a sub-genre of solo TTRPGs, which allow the player to interact and progress the story by journaling and through their own reflections.

Because of the wide variety of themes, genres, and play styles, TTRPGs have grown in popularity and often foster a sense of community. Due to the collaborative nature of TTRPGs, many communities and subcultures have developed to connect players. For example, there has been an increase in gaming conventions centered around TTRPGs, as well as a rise in popularity of hosting TTRPG nights at local stores, libraries, and other community settings. Inherently, TTRPGs work to foster connection and community among players. In the case of the COVID-19 pandemic, many sought out TTRPGs through websites such as Roll20, DnD Beyond, and Discord as a way to connect with others during a time of unprecedented isolation. This surge in popularity and increased use as a coping mechanism has resulted in the exploration of how TTRPGs can be used therapeutically.

## Ptsd

PTSD is characterized by intrusive thoughts/memories, avoidance of places, things, or even thoughts related to the event, experiences of hopelessness, numbing, and changes in physical and emotional reactions to stressors. When examining trauma, there are two kinds that can happen: experienced (primary) and vicarious (secondary). What this means is that the trauma can be experienced first hand by an individual, or it can also be witnessed, have occurred to a close friend or family member, or stem from repeated or extreme exposure to specifics regarding the event. In both cases, symptoms of PTSD can develop and impact the individual.

As a result of these symptoms, it is common for individuals who have experienced trauma(s) or been diagnosed with PTSD to become isolated from others. They may find it difficult to feel secure or safe. They may also face traumatization or have symptoms increase due to triggered events. When examining how this plays out in TTRPGs, an individual may struggle to connect with the group or character they have created. There may be an increased need to develop healthy coping, improve distress tolerance, and improve resiliency before incorporating TTRPGs.

This chapter and the case study presented serve to examine how TTRPGs can be used in the treatment of PTSD when working with individuals. TTRPGs can be utilized and incorporated therapeutically with children, teens, and adults. By incorporating TTRPGs and narratives, individuals are able to process and explore themes that may otherwise be difficult to address through more traditional modalities such as pure cognitive behavioral therapy (CBT) or psychodynamic therapy.

## PSYCHOLOGICAL IMPACT OF TRAUMA

Previously, the word trauma was most often associated with near-death experiences, loss of life or limb, and witnessing acts of violence. In modern times, there is a better understanding that trauma and traumatic experiences are much broader than these specific instances and include how the individual internalizes the experience (Griffin, 2020). Rather than focusing on whether risk of harm was evident, treatment includes whether the individual believed that risk to be real. For example, imagine a child being taken to a hospital for a high fever. Even if this is not a life-threatening illness, the experience can be traumatic from the perspective of the child who does not have the knowledge and experience to understand whether or not they are at risk of death. Several other factors can influence the severity of trauma such as if the child was abruptly separated from their caregiver, if the medical team was aggressive or obtrusive, and how the adults surrounding the child expressed their own affect and emotions. By expanding our view to examine broader traumas such as the COVID-19 pandemic, exposure to school shooting coverage, car accidents, and other experiences unique to contemporary childhood, we are better able to examine how traumatic experiences can impact an individual, how symptoms can manifest in their daily life, and how PTSD can develop.

Along with examining how we view and approach trauma, it is also crucial to address our understanding of what coping tools look like. Over time, understanding of what coping tools are and how to effectively use them has evolved.

One such evolution has been the examination of escapism. Escapism focuses on the idea of distracting oneself and is often done through various forms of entertainment such as books, movies, and theatrical productions. Similarly, TTRPGs can work to create fictitious worlds that provide a means of escapism and distraction from everyday life. By creating stories and designing characters, players are able to live vicariously through the characters they create.

In the TTRPG community, there are the concepts of "bleed in" and "bleed out." Individuals can overidentify, or "bleed in," with a character; the boundaries between the person and the character are blurred. Inversely, individuals can develop too much separation from the character they create and under-identify or "other" their character. This is an example of "bleed out." In both cases, there is an emphasis on how much players connect with their character and the ability to self-reflect as a result. Within the therapeutic setting, when using TTRPGs there must be training to look for these instances of "bleed in" or "bleed out" to further examine manifestations of trauma through how a player interacts and/or identifies with their character.

## CURRENT APPROACHES TO ADDRESSING TRAUMA

Existing research focuses on the use of individual therapy and group therapy to treat PTSD symptoms (Humble et al., 2019; Jensen et al., 2022; Mavranezouli et al., 2020b; Woollett et al., 2020). Modalities such as CBT have been used in both forms of psychotherapy. CBT focuses on altering behaviors by challenging one's assumptions, beliefs, and thought patterns (Varrette et al., 2022). Using this modality, clinicians can provide psychoeducation, promote cognitive restructuring, and develop relapse prevention. CBT has evolved to incorporate a trauma-focused approach leading to the advent of trauma-focused cognitive behavioral therapy (TF-CBT) to address PTSD specifically.

Woollett et al. (2020) found when TF-CBT is combined with art and play therapy, there is a reduction in the levels of depression in children who have witnessed domestic violence. Those involved in the study stated that art and play therapy helped them manage challenging behaviors. This study demonstrated a positive effect when working in a group; one that includes the opportunity for self-expression and working with others to address their trauma helped them see that they were not alone in the process. Group therapy helped confront the stigma and discrimination associated with the violence they have experienced (Woollett et al., 2020).

## THERAPEUTIC TABLETOP ROLEPLAYING GAMES

While TTRPGs have been around since the 1970s, they have experienced a resurgence in pop culture and the collective social consciousness in the past decade. With the rise in popularity of television shows such as Stranger

Things, the Critical Role podcast, and even celebrities discussing their experiences with TTRPGs, these games have gained renewed popularity and interest. TTRPGs have been used to connect socially with others and to communicate our stories. The rise in interest has led to the exploration of how to integrate TTRPGs therapeutically to connect with individuals through their interest in roleplaying games across developmental stages and in a variety of treatment modalities.

Varrette et al. (2022) found that when CBT was incorporated with TTRPGs in treating social anxiety in adults, there was an increased ability to explore plot points related to social anxiety and provide exposure in a measured and safe environment. Common themes illustrated through the study demonstrated the benefits of gaming in overcoming anxiety, improving social skills, and clinically connecting to their roleplay characters.

Eruyar and Vostanis (2020) illustrate the current and future potential of play therapy and gaming through their exploration of Theraplay as an intervention that can reduce PTSD-related symptoms in children diagnosed with PTSD. This approach is designed to be used in individual psychotherapy and in various settings such as residential facilities, schools, or group psychotherapy. Theraplay is an attachment-focused play therapy approach that targets six core aspects: emotional regulation, self-confidence, attachment relationships, a sense of belonging, and trust with others. Additionally, Theraplay works to include familial support figures in the therapeutic process (Eruyar & Vostanis, 2020). This modality can utilize nonverbal communication, various group activities, and games that serve to aid clients in reaching their therapeutic objectives. Utilizing the core aspects of Theraplay, clinicians are able to create opportunities to engage with the client in nurturing ways. This can provide a sense of challenge while working to increase structure. TTRPGs, like any other games, can be adapted for and integrated with the Theraplay protocol.

Group psychotherapy has long since been used to allow for the creation of community and the processing of experiences. Typically, group psychotherapy is explored as a therapeutic option once the individual is able to return to or develop a sense of safety and feels that they are able to explore experiences and topics related to past traumas with others. With this in mind, TTRPGs can be used as a tool in therapeutic settings and can be incorporated with different therapeutic modalities. The goal of therapeutic roleplaying groups is to create an environment where individuals can process and interact with past traumas in a safe way to move toward integration and cohesion. The use of roleplaying games in a therapeutic setting allows the individual to create a safe space where they can freely utilize coping tools explored in therapy while also having a degree of separation from situations encountered in the roleplay to allow further processing. Gifford (2020) suggests that therapists should look at roleplaying games (and books) as an opportunity for clients to work alongside and process their experiences with a therapist through dialogue, play therapy, and journaling. By creating and living out stories, individuals are able to develop decision-making skills in an environment that allows for trial and error in a safer way.

## INTEGRATING TTRPGS IN TRAUMA WORK WITH GROUPS

When examining treatment interventions and modalities for PTSD, a crucial component is creating safety and security. Many interventions work to establish safety and effective coping techniques before proceeding with processing memories. There are several evidence-based therapeutic approaches that are helpful in this process. Dialectical Behavioral Therapy (DBT) focuses on building distress tolerance in the beginning stages of therapy to establish safety and build resiliency. Eye Movement Desensitization and Reprocessing (EMDR) is helpful as one of the first steps that includes resourcing strategies to establish a safety anchor that the individual can use when reprocessing experiences. Similarly, there are various safety tools that have been developed for TTRPGs to empower players and give agency over themes and topics included in the roleplay.

Developing a trauma-focused integrative mindset within therapy is important when developing a therapeutic environment built on the creation of comfort, safety, and trust. Ensuring safety and trust with an individual allows for the processing and relieving of painful emotions through the implementation of evidence-based interventions (Evans, 2021; Humble et al., 2019). The development of such an environment can lead to feelings of hope and social connectedness, and the opportunity to process traumatic material and return to a pre-trauma developmental level of functioning. Due to the nature of themes, both conscious and unconscious, that can be explored through roleplay, utilizing a trauma-focused mindset allows for safety to be established and minimizes re-traumatization during the process.

Group therapy allows for connection and catharsis through the ability to share experiences with others. In a group setting, there is the opportunity to implement and develop safety tools in a collaborative way. Safety tools are established parameters and ground rules that guide how a session is conducted. They can take on different forms, such as what to do when experiencing heightened emotions, topics that are uncomfortable or to be avoided, how to express issues within the group, as well as how to respect those who are speaking. By working together to establish safety tools, rapport can be established while also building trust within the group to ensure that the space is supportive and safe for processing experiences in the future.

In the realm of TTRPGS, there are various themes and topics that may be upsetting. The use of safety tools allows for the participants and the person running the game (GM) to establish a set of ground rules regarding topics and situations that may appear in the roleplay, as well as what to do if a situation that someone is uncomfortable with should arise. One such tool that is often used in TTRPG settings is referred to as "lines and veils." The purpose of using lines and veils is to allow individuals to specify the topics and experiences they want to be excluded or reduced in their experience. A line serves as a firm boundary the individual places for a topic or experience they do not wish to have included in the roleplay. A veil, on the other hand, refers to a topic or experience that is okay to have alluded to in the roleplay but not experienced directly. For example, if an individual identifies spiders as a line, this means they are not comfortable having spiders in the roleplay by any means. However, if the individual identifies spiders as a veil, then it is okay to allude to the fact that spiders exist by mentioning a cobweb, but no spiders would be encountered in the roleplay.

When utilizing TTRPGs in a therapeutic setting, whether it is a group or individual, creating and maintaining safety in the session is crucial. By incorporating these tools during the formation of the group, safety is established by having clear boundaries and rules that can continue to be reinforced going forward. As the roleplay proceeds, themes and situations can be explored in a measured and controlled way. Through this process, group members are able to acknowledge possible triggers for painful memories or increases in symptoms related to PTSD in a non-judgmental format. Lines and veils can always be revisited to ensure that the safety of individuals and the group is reinforced, while also allowing for possible topics to be explored in individual settings as well, if necessary.

When working with adult individuals, themes and topics explored in TTRPGs may be more complex. This can lead to more challenging themes such as death, grief, and relationship conflict, as well as others to be explored. Because these themes may be more mature than would be the case when working with children and adolescents, the need for safety tools to prevent re-traumatization during the roleplay is vital. While safety tools are necessary when establishing a group of any age, establishing ground rules for conduct in the roleplay, as well as how to communicate when an individual is uncomfortable, allows those participating to proceed with more ease of mind. This is especially the case when examining if TTRPGs are an appropriate therapeutic tool for an individual or group.

## CASE EXAMPLE

Golgotha, a 31-year-old adult, was referred to therapy after stepping down from a therapeutic group home and returning to the community. The client and family reported a diagnostic history of trauma, autism, and intermittent explosive disorder. Additionally, Golgotha reported struggling with stress management and often feeling overwhelmed. His family indicated during the intake that a lack of effective coping techniques exacerbated the current concerns. The client experienced several ongoing chronic medical conditions contributing to his behaviors, including ongoing risk of seizures, neuropathy of the colon that required an implant to reduce fecal incontinence, and a history of idiopathic growth hormone disorder. The client's experience of chronic ongoing traumas was associated with his history of aggression toward others, inability to control emotions, witnessing violence in the home, and being attacked in the group home. The client reported sustaining an organic brain injury from one of the multiple attacks within his previous group placement. Golgotha had a history of being physically aggressive toward his mother and sister before placement within an adult group home. Although the client is now residing in independent living, his mother is his legal guardian and power of attorney. His mother arranges all services the client receives to stay in the community.

During the intake appointment, it was reported that during his childhood, Golgotha had been a witness to violence in the home by his father against his mother. The interpersonal violence experienced in the home resulted in Golgotha becoming violent with his mother as well, serving as a generational cascade for the family system. At the beginning of therapy, Golgotha's mood and behaviors were volatile. At times, he presented as withdrawn and quiet. At other times, he would engage in explosive anger with Golgotha yelling and trying to intimidate the clinician. Golgotha's primary treatment goal was to remain in the community. Over time, he began working on taking personal responsibility and accountability for his actions to achieve this goal.

One of the ways Golgotha and his father connected while he was in residential care was while playing Dungeons and Dragons (DnD). This resulted in Golgotha having an emotional connection with TTRPGs. Shortly before beginning outpatient therapy services, an incident took place where Golgotha had been participating in a DnD campaign with his father and some support staff. However, all the staff quit at the same time, which resulted in Golgotha losing both the connections to his attachment figures in the residential setting and the quality time with his father. This resulted in the physical game of DnD becoming a trigger for increased anxiety and other PTSD-related symptoms due to the sudden loss. Despite this event being a source of increased anxiety and distress for Golgotha, he still wanted to utilize DnD in his therapy sessions and participate in a roleplaying group immediately upon beginning services. For Golgotha, DnD was seen as one of the few ways he knew to connect with others, and he wanted to regain the positive experience.

After the intake, Golgotha took part in four individual sessions where he was assessed for appropriateness in joining a therapeutic group. In the early sessions, Golgotha's communication skills were limited. While he was fully verbal, he often lacked the ability to convey the ideas and themes he wanted to address effectively. In short, he had a story he wanted to tell but not the means to tell it. Upon observing this, play was introduced into individual sessions through board games and the use of a different TTRPG, Numinera. By changing the TTRPG being played, the opportunity for change was presented through this new system. After four individual sessions, Golgotha was incorporated into a therapeutic roleplaying group where he continued to use the Numinera system to tell stories.

This therapeutic group was designed to increase emotional regulation and enhance the social navigation needs of the participants. While trauma was not the main focus of the group, each of the participating members had past traumatic experiences that they were working to process through individual sessions as well. Originally, Golgotha had a very domineering play style in the roleplay. He would often dictate what other group members were doing on their turn, thus removing their personal agency from the gameplay. Over time, he was able to work to become more collaborative and co-creative to create a story with the other group members rather than acting out his own.

Golgotha demonstrated difficulty connecting with others in the group and acted out in a form of solo play where he was the narrator of the story being told. Many of the characters that he created were half-mechanized or half-inorganic. Golgotha often designed characters that struggled socially but sought connection with others. Through his roleplay, the theme of "becoming whole" was often acted out.

After roughly 3–6 months of participating in individual and group therapy sessions, DnD was reintroduced as part of individual psychotherapy. DnD was used as a solo-journaling experience where Golgotha was challenged to push against his tendency to dictate the actions of others and control others in play. DnD served as a successful tool in enhancing Golgotha's social navigation and reduced his micromanaging of others. In recent sessions, the reduction in symptoms related to PTSD has resulted in Golgotha's ability to shift the focus of his therapeutic goals toward developing and understanding attachments. He initiates the focus on examining relationships, boundaries, and unhealthy patterns within relationships to develop enhanced connections with others. There have been no reports of explosive anger in the last 6 months, and Golgotha has maintained his ability to live on his own within the community.

## CONSIDERATIONS FOR THE USE OF THERAPEUTIC TABLETOP GAMEPLAY IN RESEARCH AND PRACTICE

There is evidence to suggest that the use of play-based techniques such as TTRPGs can aid in the reduction of trauma symptoms (Evans, 2020). Research suggests that TF-CBT and, to a lesser degree, play therapy are effective ways to treat PTSD in youth (Mavranezouli et al., 2020a). If that is the case, then exploratory studies should focus on combining these different approaches, using one to inform the other (Mavranezouli et al., 2020a).

Within the intersection of therapeutic modalities, gameplay, and trauma, it is important for clinicians to try to "meet" clients where they are developmentally and emotionally. There is a need for therapists to understand their clients' insight into their lifestyles through direct/indirect teaching and metaphorical transfer (Ashby et al., 2020). In their research focused on Adlerian Play Therapy and Adventure Therapy, Ashby et al. (2020) discuss how additional types of resilience can come from the courage present in a child demonstrated through their experience and the child's belief that they can face psychological risks without a guarantee of success. This highlights the need for therapeutic settings to allow for experiential play to develop necessary coping and build resilience that may otherwise be difficult to address.

When selecting game-based interventions, a clinician should consider how that gameplay can lead to mastery of transferable skills (Fonzo et al., 2019; Kühn et al., 2014). It is crucial to ensure that game-based interventions are still evidence-based and that the game selected matches both the therapeutic approach and the themes being addressed in the session. This is especially true when utilizing TTRPGs due to the vast themes, mechanics, and topics that can be addressed. These factors are also why it is important to utilize safety tools. Too often, practitioners ask how to use a given game in the session rather than if they should. By further developing evidence-based interventions, practitioners will be better prepared to understand the concerns that can be addressed through the use of TTRPGs and gauge the appropriateness for the individuals they work with.

Future research can compare trauma-informed modalities that incorporate TTRPGs with control groups to see if the efficacy of these modalities differs from other trauma-focused interventions (Evans, 2021). Some of these studies would benefit from varying the duration of treatment and incorporating repeated affective, cognitive, and symptom assessments throughout to determine optimal patterns and to isolate better specific mechanisms of symptom change (Fonzo et al., 2019). There is a need for further research on these techniques when applied to both digital and non-digital gameplay therapy.

If we start by creating feasibility studies, we can better understand if a given intervention and measure work with target populations (Eruyar & Vostanis, 2020). A small pilot study can test all the components of an intervention, allowing a large-scale study that examines the effectiveness of the intervention. As the research suggests, novel treatment options that clients find engaging are needed to address the ongoing public healthcare issues associated with PTSD (Butler et al., 2020; Fonzo et al., 2019; Kühn et al., 2014).

Furthermore, it is necessary to understand the limitations of such approaches and their use. There is a need for safety mechanics, tools, theories, and interventions to aid clients in empathizing character-personas and narrative forms that they may emulate through gameplay while mentally reimagining themselves through TTRPG worlds (Gifford, 2020).

Clients need opportunities to find healing in fiction, fantasy, and self-expression. Additionally, there is a need to understand the nature of emotional regulation and actively involve parents, caregivers, and other individuals who support our clients' lives (Eruyar & Vostanis, 2020; Woollett et al., 2020). Exploratory qualitative research is needed to focus on the relationship between caregivers and children as they attempt to work through shared trauma and abuse. There is a need to compare gameplay (digital and TTRPGs) with other forms of therapeutic interventions in both qualitative and quantitative individual and group studies. The goal is to develop new ways to help clients exercise healthy adaptive skills that lead to social and relational connections (Varrette et al., 2022). Future studies can look to understand the causal effects between interventions and trauma (Evans, 2021). Through exploring therapeutic applications of gameplay, we may find new alternatives to aid clients in developing resiliency to address symptomatology associated with post-traumatic stress.

## CONCLUSION

A trauma-informed integrative approach utilizing TTRPGs in gameplay therapy can lead to various emotional responses. The opportunity for self-exploration through TTRPGs can foster emotional growth and well-being through re-evaluating one's traumas and how they can irreparably change one's perceived identity and the catharsis that comes with acceptance. It is worth noting that understanding game design's influence on how a client engages during the therapeutic process is essential. As with any toy, tool, game system, or intervention, a therapist is ethically responsible for understanding how the use of a game impacts the opportunity for therapeutic change. TTRPGs can provide an opportunity to explore one's trauma by evaluating the pain and trauma associated with those outside oneself. In a sense, TTRPGs can serve as a mirror to allow individuals the opportunity to examine their experience from another perspective. The use of TTRPGs in the therapeutic setting can foster opportunities for reflection by adding a degree of separation when examining situations. As clinicians, it is our responsibility to aid clients in identifying and interpreting the impact that trauma has had on themselves and those around them.

## REFERENCES

Ashby, J. S., Tobin, G. K., & Mi Kyoung, J. (2020). Adlerian play therapy and adventure therapy: Complementary interventions for comprehensive theory. *Journal of Individual Psychology*, 76(2), 187–200. https://doi-org.unioncc.idm.oclc.org/10.1353/jip.2020.0000

Butler, O., Herr, K., Willmund, G., Gallinat, J., Kühn, S., & Zimmermann, P. (2020). Trauma, treatment, and Tetris: video gaming increases hippocampal volume in male patients with combat-related post-traumatic stress disorder. *Journal of Psychiatry & Neuroscience*, 45(4), 279–287. https://doi-org.unioncc.idm.oclc.org/10.1503/jpn.190027

Eruyar, S., & Vostanis, P. (2020). Feasibility of group therapy with refugee children in Turkey. *Counselling and Psychotherapy Research*, 20(4), 626–637. https://doi-org.unioncc.idm.oclc.org/10.1002/capr.12354

Evans, C. (2020). Adlerian play therapy and trauma. *Journal of Individual Psychology*, 76(2), 217–228. https://doi-org.unioncc.idm.oclc.org/10.1353/jip.2020.0002

Evans, C. (2021). Trauma-informed Adlerian play therapy: A case study. *Journal of Individual Psychology*, 77(3), 362–373. https://doi-org.unioncc.idm.oclc.org/10.1353/jip.2021.0025

Fonzo, G. A., Fine, N. B., Wright, R. N., Achituv, M., Zaiko, Y. V., Merin, O., Shalev, A. Y., & Etkin, A. (2019). Internet-delivered computerized cognitive & affective remediation training for the treatment of acute and chronic post-traumatic stress disorder: Two randomized clinical trials. *Journal of Psychiatric Research*, 115, 82–89. https://doi-org.unioncc.idm.oclc.org/10.1016/j.jpsychires.2019.05.007

Gifford, J. (2020). Roleplaying, reader response, and play-therapy in fantasy fiction: "You could hear the dice rolling" in novels about abuse and recovery. *English Studies in Canada*, 46(1), 1–28. https://doi-org.unioncc.idm.oclc.org/10.1353/esc.2020.0000

Griffin, G. (2020). Defining trauma and a trauma-informed COVID-19 response. *Psychological Trauma Theory Research Practice and Policy*, 12(S1), S279–S280. https://doi.org/10.1037/tra0000828

Humble, J. J., Summers, N. L., Villarreal, V., Styck, K. M., Sullivan, J. R., Hechler, J. M., & Warren, B. S. (2019). Child-centered play therapy for youths who have experienced trauma: A systematic literature review. *Journal of Child & Adolescent Trauma*, 12(3), 365–375. https://doi-org.unioncc.idm.oclc.org/10.1007/s40653-018-0235-7

Jensen, T. K., Braathu, N., Birkeland, M. S., Ormhaug, S. M., & Skar, A. S. (2022). Complex PTSD and treatment outcomes in TF-CBT for youth: A naturalistic study. *European Journal of Psychotraumatology*, 13(2), 2114630. https://doi.org/10.1080/20008066.2022.2114630

Kühn, S., Gleich, T., Lorenz, R. C., Lindenberger, U., & Gallinat, J. (2014). Playing Super Mario induces structural brain plasticity: Gray matter changes resulting from training with a commercial video game. *Molecular Psychiatry*, 19(2), 272. https://doi-org.unioncc.idm.oclc.org/10.1038/mp.2013.120

Mavranezouli, I., Megnin, V. O., Daly, C., Dias, S., Stockton, S., Meiser, S. R., Trickey, D., & Pilling, S. (2020a). Research review: Psychological and psychosocial treatments for children and young people with post-traumatic stress disorder: A network meta-analysis. *Journal of Child Psychology & Psychiatry*, 61(1), 18–29. https://doi-org.unioncc.idm.oclc.org/10.1111/jcpp.13094

Mavranezouli, I., Megnin, V. O., Trickey, D., Meiser, S. R., Daly, C., Dias, S., Stockton, S., & Pilling, S. (2020b). Cost-effectiveness of psychological interventions for children and young people with post-traumatic stress disorder. *Journal of Child Psychology & Psychiatry, 61*(6), 699–710. https://doi-org.unioncc.idm.oclc.org/10.1111/jcpp.13142

Sloan, D. M., Bovin, M. J., & Schnurr, P. P. (2012). Review of group treatment for PTSD. *Journal of Rehabilitation Research and Development, 49*(5), 689–701. https://doi.org/10.1682/jrrd.2011.07.0123

Woollett, N., Bandeira, M., & Hatcher, A. (2020). Trauma-informed art and play therapy: Pilot study outcomes for children and mothers in domestic violence shelters in the United States and South Africa. *Child Abuse & Neglect, 107*, N.PAG. https://doi-org.unioncc.idm.oclc.org/10.1016/j.chiabu.2020.104564

Varrette, M., Berkenstock, J., Greenwood-Ericksen, A., Ortega, A., Michaels, F., Pietrobon, V., & Schodorf, M. (2022). Exploring the efficacy of cognitive behavioral therapy and roleplaying games as an intervention for adults with social anxiety. *Social Work with Groups*, 1–17. https://doi.org/10.1080/01609513.2022.2146029

## CHAPTER SEVENTEEN

# Social Media and Trauma

KRISTINE J. DOTY-YELLS and DAVID P. YELLS

Social media use (SMU) has become a global staple of life. People can be seen absorbed in their cell phones, whether they are walking down a street, dining with family or friends, or even working at their jobs. The possession of cell phones and other electronic devices dominates life, and most users are engaging with at least one social media (SM) platform. This chapter will explore how the perceived need for SM impacts multiple aspects of our daily living and creates societal shifts.

SM is ubiquitous in modern life. Statista (2022) reports 4.59 billion SM users in 2022, up 1 billion from 2019. They project another billion SM users by 2025. Pew Research Center (2021) reported that most American adults use SM. More than half of adults visit at least one SM site daily. The two most popular sites by far are YouTube, used by 81% of adults, and Facebook, used by 69%. There are nine other SM sites that are popular among adults (see Table 17.1).

Many adults over 65 use Facebook and some use YouTube, but few older adults use other sites (Pew Research Center, 2021). There are platforms designed for specific populations, such as LinkedIn, Pinterest, and NextDoor. LinkedIn is a career platform targeted toward educated and business-minded people. Pinterest, favored by women, is a creative platform used to share ideas and images. Neighbors connect, share local news and events, and report criminal activity or lost pets through NextDoor.

Cell phone use is naturally correlated with SMU. Pew Research Center (2021) reports 87% of all Americans own a smartphone. However, that number

*Trauma Impacts: The Repercussions of Individual and Collective Trauma*, First Edition.
Edited by Jessica Stone, Robert J. Grant, and Clair Mellenthin.
© 2024 John Wiley & Sons, Inc. Published 2024 by John Wiley & Sons, Inc.

**Table 17.1**
Social Media Sites by Adult Use

| Social media site | Percentage of adults using site |
| --- | --- |
| Instagram | 40 |
| Pinterest | 31 |
| LinkedIn | 28 |
| Snapchat | 25 |
| Twitter | 23 |
| WhatsApp | 23 |
| TikTok | 21 |
| Reddit | 18 |
| NextDoor | 13 |

**Table 17.2**
Social Media Sites by Teen Use

| Social media site | Percentage of teens using site |
| --- | --- |
| YouTube | 77 |
| TikTok | 58 |
| Snapchat | 51 |
| Instagram | 50 |
| Facebook | 19 |

increases to 96% when considering adults ages 18–49. Adolescents and children are obtaining cell phones at increasingly younger ages, and they quickly discover the ease and convenience of connecting with friends and family through SM. Younger adults, ages 18–30, primarily use Instagram, Snapchat, and TikTok.

Another Pew Research Center study (2022a) regarding SMU via teens ages 13–17 indicates 97% use of the internet almost daily, while 46% use it almost constantly. There are five SM platforms that are the most popular among teens (Table 17.2).

It is worth noting, and perhaps alarming, that more than one-third of teens are on one of these sites almost constantly (Pew Research Center, 2022a). Unfortunately, there are no published studies regarding SMU by children. It is unknown at what age children first access SM, which platforms they use, and how much time they spend using it.

## SOCIAL MEDIA IN THE MAINSTREAM MEDIA

SM is often the subject of news stories in mainstream media. Over the past few years, much of the news regarding SM has been negative. For example, Facebook has been criticized regularly. It was fined $725 million for data privacy violations (NBC News, 2022). It has been the subject of congressional investigations (CNN Business, 2021) regarding, among other issues, harmful effects on teenage users. More recently, TikTok has been condemned because of concerns regarding information security (CBS News, 2022).

## BENEFITS OF SOCIAL MEDIA USE

SMU has been criticized for its negative effects; however, what is often not reported are the potential mental health benefits. There is support that SMU may have positive effects on mental health. A body of evidence has emerged which suggests people have used SM to cope with primary and secondary traumatic experiences. SMU can be credited for helping people stay connected to friends and family. Additionally, SM helps people with similar interests and circumstances find mutual support.

### INFORMATION DISSEMINATION

Zhong et al. (2021) examined SMU among Wuhan residents at the peak of the COVID-19 pandemic. Results indicated that residents used SM to gather valuable information. They also reported significant peer and emotional support by accessing and sharing health information about the situation. Access to information is an important factor mitigating the effects of trauma, such as an emerging public health crisis.

The American Red Cross is an organization that provides important services in emergency assistance and disaster relief (American Red Cross, n.d.). The Red Cross is a good example of an organization that leverages SM to help individuals dealing with trauma from a variety of sources (e.g., natural disasters, terrorism, and war). Research on its use of SM (Briones et al., 2011) has focused on building relationships, which can be vital in mitigating the effects of trauma. For example, the Red Cross can spread word of the existence of a disaster situation, engage donors, and recruit volunteers to assist in its efforts. Additionally, during a natural disaster, it maintains an SM site where survivors can report their status to worried family members and friends.

### FINDING AND MAINTAINING CONNECTION

Another study (Zhen et al., 2021) examined the effects of SMU on U.S. college students during the COVID-19 pandemic. In particular, the authors were interested in the role of self-disclosure on SM. They distinguished between peripheral self-disclosure and core self-disclosure. The former refers to general information that individuals share widely on SM, whereas the latter refers to more limited private information that individuals share with close friends only. Results indicated that core self-disclosure was associated with a reduction in perceived stress resulting from disruptions in life due to COVID-19, thereby reducing the potential for trauma.

Another common source of stress and trauma is acculturation. International students are subject to significant acculturation stress and more than 5% of the U.S. higher education population are international students. Li and Peng (2019) explored the use of SM in moderating acculturation stress in this population. They reported that SMU with the host and home country was associated with less acculturation stress.

## Emotional Support through Traumatic Experiences

Researchers have also investigated the use of SM in situations of a more personal nature. For example, Hoffman et al. (2021) explored the use of SM by individuals who had experienced the loss of a loved one. Participants reported that SM was moderately helpful in dealing with their loss. Specific benefits of SM use included useful dissemination of information, general support, and the ability to share memories.

Cristall et al. (2021) explored the use of SM among individuals with severe burn injuries. They focused on the sharing of burn narratives posted on survivor-patient websites. Severe burn injuries are acutely traumatic and leave long-lasting physical and emotional scars. These web-based platforms provide a valuable opportunity for patients to share their experiences and receive support.

People with a common purpose can connect with others online. "Hashtag activism" allows people with a shared experience to find each other and discuss specific elements of their trauma that may be difficult to share in person, such as sexual trauma. One well-known example is the #MeToo movement, where women who were sexually harassed united under this hashtag to share their experiences and publicize it as a widespread problem. Whiting et al. (2021) analyzed a group of tweets under the hashtag #WhyIDidntReport to evaluate the reasons victims did not report their sexual assault. Respondents included men and women who shared specific and often deeply personal reasons they chose not to report. The ability to remain anonymous made it easier for them to disclose this information. They found a shared camaraderie with others who endured this traumatic experience.

## Financial and Institutional Support

Levaot et al. (2021) focused their research on adults who experienced large-scale fires in Israel in 2016. Their measures included questionnaires on giving and receiving offers of assistance via SM, along with checklists for post-traumatic stress and post-traumatic growth. Their results indicated that use of SM for giving or receiving offers of assistance was positively associated with post-traumatic growth, such as increased personal strength and appreciation of life. There was no relationship between the use of SM and post-traumatic stress.

Dealing with trauma resulting from natural disasters is another case of the potential value of SM. McKay and Perez (2019) studied the aftermath of Typhoon Haiyan in the Philippines. They emphasized the role of "citizen aid," the assistance provided by local and informal groups to fellow citizens on the front line of a disaster. This assistance is often facilitated by brokers; actors who unite and assist in exchanges among various entities. McKay and Perez (2019) highlighted the importance of SM (Facebook) in this process. They found that using SM to circulate images was helpful in raising funds to support aid efforts. Although this study did not include any direct measures of trauma, it is reasonable to assume that their efforts contributed to a reduction in trauma among the residents affected by the typhoon.

## Social Media and Mental Health: Positives

Hampton (2019) investigated the effect of using SM and other computer technologies on changes in psychological distress and severe psychological distress over time. The sample for his study came from the Panel Study of Income Dynamics, the longest-running longitudinal household panel survey. Participants completed the K6, a measure of psychological distress. He found that the use of SM, in combination with general internet use, contributed to reduced psychological distress. Moreover, the use of SM significantly reduced the risk of serious psychological distress. Specifically, the use of SM was only slightly less effective than in-person social contact in lessening the likelihood of severe psychological distress.

The use of SM in less extreme forms of trauma such as loneliness and attachment disorder has also been investigated (Benoit & DiTommaso, 2020). Attachment insecurity can result in increased loneliness, which is associated with a host of negative mental health outcomes. Perceived social support can attenuate the relationship between attachment insecurity and loneliness. Benoit and DiTommaso (2020) reported that online perceived social support served to mediate the relationship between attachment avoidance and chronic social loneliness, as well as the relationship between attachment anxiety and chronic social loneliness. In other words, individuals with insecure attachment may find relief from experiencing loneliness by taking advantage of SM as a form of social support.

Bekalu et al. (2019) conducted a more nuanced assessment of the impact of SM usage on mental health. They examined both the extent of SMU, as well as the users' level of emotional connection. They found routine use of SM was positively associated with social well-being, positive mental health, and self-rated health. However, they also found that higher levels of emotional connection to SM were negatively associated with those same measures.

Prescott et al. (2020) explored the explicit use of SM in a mental health context. They studied the use of an Online Mental Health Community (OMHC), which is a chat room that allows users to share personal experiences regarding their mental health. Their research indicated that users relied on the OMHC for both emotional and informational support. The researchers also suggest that OMHCs have the potential to increase self-efficacy among users, which may help them transition to further support.

## DETRIMENTS OF SOCIAL MEDIA USE

While there are many benefits of SMU, it would be irresponsible not to include a discussion of the potential problems associated with its use.

### Incivility, Division, and Violence

SM sites promote the use of *groups* and *pages* for people who share a common interest. As discussed above, these groups are often created for sharing experiences and garnering social support. However, not all groups exist for such a purpose. An increasing number of radical political organizations are using SM to further their violent or extremist views. Some of them begin by uniting in a shared purpose or ideology, such as political viewpoints, social activism, and shared opinions, but then they turn dark and insidious. Stroinska and Cecchetto (2019) explained sometimes extremist groups will support other groups with similar goals and purposes and unite to oppose people and groups who represent different ideals and purposes. They may use "codes" to post obscure messages to people meant to understand them and take action. When such groups target "other" groups based on religious, racial, ethnic traits, or political viewpoints, the result can be open expression and promotion of hate speech. On a national or global scale, one group may blame "the other" for social or political ills. As such thought is broadcast at the speed of SM, people are influenced by such opinions, especially when they are projected as facts. The political and social divide widens, and "the other" becomes anyone with whom you disagree. This is especially dangerous when such groups attract or attack vulnerable people. We are now observing the increasing tendency to use uncivil language and degrade "the other" throughout the world (Stroinska & Cecchetto, 2019). The ability to promote ideas anonymously has made incivility much easier. We say things about and to people on SM that we may never say to them in person. This leads to a more microlevel problem, that of cyberbullying.

Cyberbullying

Cyberbullying is "using computers or other information technology devices…
to embarrass, harass, intimidate, threaten, or otherwise cause harm to individuals targeted for such abuse" (McQuade III et al., 2009, p. ix). SM provides
a convenient and accessible environment for the perpetuation of cyberbullying. It is an opportune place for people who want to remain anonymous to
feel emboldened to bully others, particularly through rumors and hate speech.
Rumors can spread within seconds online, and reputations can be ruined in a
matter of hours.

SM platforms such as TikTok and Facebook are used to post photos and
videos of bullying, fighting, and other aggressive and abusive behaviors. This
can be humiliating for all those involved. Videos circulate and become fuel
for shaming and embarrassment. Often, the sharing of these videos is cycli-
cal, causing multiple rounds of degradation. In clinical practice, one of the
authors saw a teen boy who complained of such bullying. He said people
have brought up stories and mistakes of his from several years back and
repeatedly circulated them on SM to embarrass him. He said he cannot get
past the foolish behavior of his elementary school years because the old posts
seemed to come back to haunt him.

Bullying perpetrators who are already traumatized from childhood experiences are particularly vulnerable to the misuse of SM. Kircaburun et al. (2020)
discovered that childhood trauma is both a direct and indirect predictor of
the perpetration of cyberbullying by college-age students. This same study
also indicated that childhood trauma is associated with the development of
narcissistic, antisocial, and borderline personality traits, which in turn, are
also associated with cyberbullying. The authors suggest it is important for
clinicians to consider assessing for personality disorders when treating people with cyberbullying behaviors.

Social Media and Smartphone Addiction

Certainly, there are benefits to people having access to SM, but excessive use
can become problematic (Ramazanoglu, 2020). It is concerning enough that,
perhaps surprisingly, assessment tools have been created and standardized to
measure SMU, such as the Bergen Facebook Addiction Scale, the Bergen
Social Media Scale (van den Eijnden et al., 2016), and the Smartphone
Addiction Scale (Ithnain et al., 2018).

The term *addiction* when applied to the use of electronics, the internet, or
SM, is an issue under debate. There are a variety of terms used, including
problematic use, dependency, disordered use, and others. Refer to Huang
(2022) for a discussion of the terminology used in the scholarly literature.

This chapter uses *problematic use* except when the study mentioned uses other specific terms.

In their meta-analysis of research studying problematic SMU and its link with problematic smartphone use, Marino and associates (2019) found a significant relationship between smartphone addiction and problematic SMU. However, the authors suggest taking caution when evaluating the results because SM is often accessed via tablets and computers, so the exact amount of problematic SMU cannot be determined. In addition, people use their smartphones for other purposes, such as texting, watching movies, and using non-SM applications, so there may be other reasons for the problematic smartphone use. Nevertheless, negative psychological outcomes are correlated with both problematic smartphone use and problematic SMU (Marino et al., 2019).

Ithnain et al. (2018) studied college students in Malaysia to determine the link between smartphone addiction and anxiety and depression. Using the Smartphone Addiction Scale, they found more than 70% of the students used smartphones in excess of 4 hours per day. More than half used them primarily to access SM sites. Roughly half of the students studied showed high levels of smartphone addiction. The authors determined that smartphone addiction is a predictor of anxiety and depression. Ramazanoglu (2020) has suggested that smartphone and SM addiction are part of a broader addiction to technology. In his study, he found a high and significant correlation between smartphone addiction, internet use, and SM addiction.

## SOCIAL MEDIA AND MENTAL HEALTH: NEGATIVES

Huang (2022) conducted a statistical meta-analysis of 133 studies examining problematic SMU and a variety of mental health concerns across all SM platforms. The articles he analyzed used a variety of different instruments to measure problematic SMU, as well as different mental health issues. His overall findings revealed problematic SMU is negatively correlated with self-esteem and life satisfaction and positively correlated with loneliness and depression. In other words, problematic SMU is related to lower levels of self-esteem and life satisfaction and higher levels of loneliness and depression. This was particularly true in males, for whom Huang recommends targeted mental health assistance.

Sadagheyani and Tatari (2021) conducted a meta-analysis of 50 studies evaluating the impact of SM on mental health. They concluded that SMU has both negative and positive effects. The authors found positive effects that included accessing expert health information and health experiences of others, mental health resources, emotional support, connection with peers, and maintaining relationships that helped reduce depression. Negative effects include higher rates of anxiety and depression, poor quality of sleep, thoughts of self-harm, suicidal ideation, poor body image, and poor life satisfaction. It is notable that the results showed evidence for both increases and decreases in rates of depression.

Shannon et al. (2022) also performed a meta-analysis of articles regarding problematic SMU and its effect on mental health. They found a significant correlation between problematic SMU and depression, anxiety, and stress. An important consideration with all three of the meta-analyses is that they could only show a correlation; none of them could show that problematic SMU was the cause of the mental health problems.

Louragli et al. (2019) studied the impact of Facebook addiction on college students in Morocco. They found students who were addicted to Facebook had higher rates of anxiety than those who were not. The study also showed that Moroccan adolescents surveyed spend an average of 4 hours per day on their smartphones and nearly 1 hour per day on their personal computers. For more than 75% of the time spent on their smartphones, they are connected to the internet, and most of these students access SM immediately upon initial connection.

In Zhong and associates' study (2021) regarding SMU and COVID-19 in Wuhan, the results indicated that SMU significantly *predicted* depression, with higher levels of SMU being associated with more severe depression. Their analysis also revealed that SMU may predict secondary trauma, in which a person becomes distressed from learning about the traumatic experiences of others. It is not surprising that they found higher levels of SMU associated with more severe secondary trauma. First et al. (2021) found people gaining exposure to more information about COVID-19 through SM experienced more psychological distress and depression.

## Youth Attitudes of Social Media

Pew Research Center (2022b) reported that youth are generally unconcerned about their privacy and information security on SM. In the study, 60% of teens said they believed they had little to no control over the amount of their personal information that is shared with companies, and 44% indicated they had little to no concern about it. At the very least, these findings raise a potential teen safety issue.

Pew Research Center (2022b) also studied how teens believed their parents were concerned about their experiences using SM. Surprisingly, 41% of teens said their parents were not at all or not very concerned about their use, and 9% did not know how their parents felt about it, that is, half of parents are unaware of how SM is impacting their children. Teens were also asked how their parents see their SM experience. Many teens (39%) believe their experiences on SM are better than their parents think, and 27% claim they are worse.

Finally, the Pew study (2022b) revealed that nearly half of teen girls feel overwhelmed by all the drama they see on SM, 37% feel left out of things by their friends, and 28% say SM made them feel worse about their own lives.

Teens have become very SM savvy. In a CNN podcast, *Chasing Life*, host Dr. Sanjay Gupta interviewed his daughters to hear their thoughts about teen SMU. Gupta asked specifically about their opinion of the U.S. banning access to TikTok. His daughter Soleil replied, "You know what all the teenagers are going to do? They're going to set their phones so that they live in Canada. And they're still gonna use Snapchat and TikTok" (Gupta, 2023).

We are left to wonder why so many parents are not concerned about SM. Why is there such a gap in parents' knowledge of their teen's use of SM? And perhaps most importantly, why are they not having honest discussions about what content their children are accessing and what types of interactions they are engaging in?

## RECOMMENDATIONS

Like most products of the digital age, SM is a double-edged sword. There are benefits and detriments to using it, and care and self-control should be practiced. When it comes to adolescents and children, appropriate parental monitoring, involvement, and oversight should be employed.

In terms of benefits, SM can be leveraged as a resource for mental health treatment, as reported by Prescott et al. (2020). In fact, the Association of American Medical Colleges (n.d.) reports that more than 150 million Americans live in federally designated mental health professional shortage areas. Judicious use of SM could help address this shortage. There are potential clients for whom the distance for face-to-face mental health care is prohibitive, and others prefer the privacy and convenience offered by internet therapy.

In March, U.S. President Joe Biden used his State of the Union address to present his national perspective and recommendations on the use of SM for youth. They include the following:

- Strengthen children's privacy and ban targeted advertising for children online
- Institute stronger online protections for young people
- Stop discriminatory algorithmic decision-making that limits opportunities for young Americans
- Invest in research on the mental harms of SM (The White House, 2022)

We would add one more recommendation: limit access to SM for youth under 18. Dr. Vivek Murthy, U.S. Surgeon General, has criticized the impact of SM on children. He suggested 13 is too young to use SM, explaining that during adolescence, "kids are developing their identity and their sense of self. . . And the skewed and often distorted environment of social media often does a disservice to many of those children" (CNN Health, 2023). We are aware banning SM for teens would not be a popular decision as, not surprisingly, 54% of teens say it would be hard or very hard to give it up (Pew Research Center, 2022a).

As a mental health practitioner, one of the authors has seen many children find themselves on SM too soon, and they are accessing material that is inappropriate for their age. Viewing such content may cause or worsen trauma. We encourage parents to band together to set community standards to guide their children's use of SM. We raise a clarion call to lawmakers, technology companies, and schools to consider the health and safety needs of children above political or economic expediency. We must create a safer experience for our children on SM.

At a bare minimum, we urge parents everywhere to learn more about SM and make their feelings about it clearly known to their children. Most importantly, parents must set limits to protect children from accessing inappropriate material and activities that will damage teens' self-esteem and safety.

We also suggest adults commit to withdrawing from all SM for 10 days as a personal test. To temporarily abstain would serve as a gauge for how much time is spent using SM, whether that use is problematic, and how changes can be made to its use. The authors have done it, and it has made a big difference. We owe it to ourselves, our children, our employers, and society to reclaim the balance in our lives, and the safety and well-being of our children by not allowing SM to rule them.

## REFERENCES

American Red Cross. (n.d.). The American National Red Cross. https://www.redcross.org/?cid=generic&med=cpc&source=google&scode=RSG00000E017&gclid=CjwKCAiAlp2fBhBPEiwA2Q10DxQ6u3ZAWt_Um2iXpUJRg1vhOxoq4XVCtaBSQCs5KgZlYy00m-iakxoCnUgQAvD_BwE&gclsrc=aw.ds

Association of American Medical Colleges. (n.d.). *A growing psychiatrist shortage and an enormous demand for mental health services.* https://www.aamc.org/news-insights/growing-psychiatrist-shortage-enormous-demand-mental-health-services

Bekalu, M. A., McCloud, R. F., & Viswanath, K. (2019). Association of social media use with social well-being, positive mental health, and self-rated health: Disentangling routine use from emotional connection to use. *Health, Education, & Behavior, 46*(25), 69S–80S.

Benoit, A., & DiTommaso, E. (2020). Attachment, loneliness, and online perceived social support. *Personality and Individual Differences, 167*, 1–7.

Briones, R. L., Kuch, B., Liu, B. F., & Jin, Y. (2011). Keeping up with the digital age: How the American Red Cross uses social media to build relationships. *Public Relations Review, 37*, 37–43.

CBS News (2022, December). *TikTok faces growing national security concerns: "It's not just the collection of theft of that data"*. https://www.cbsnews.com/news/tiktok-security-concerns-china-data/

CNN Business (2021, October). *Facebook whistleblower testifies in congress*. https://www.cnn.com/business/live-newss/facebook-senate-hearing-10-05-21/index.html

CNN Health (2023, January 29). *Surgeon general says 13 is too young to join social media*. https://www.cnn.com/2023/01/29/health/surgeon-general-social-media/index.html

Cristall, N., Kohja, Z., Gawaziuk, J. P., Spiwak, R., & Logsetty, S. (2021). Narrative discourse of burn injury and recovery on peer support websites: A qualitative analysis. *Burns, 47*(2), 397–410.

van den Eijnden, R. J. J. M., Lemmens, J. S., & Valkenburg, P. M. (2016). The social media scale. *Computers in Human Behavior, 61*, 478–487.

First, J. M., Shin, H., Ranjit, Y. S., & Houston, J. B. (2021). COVID-19 stress and depression: Examining social media, traditional media, and interpersonal communication. *Journal of Loss and Trauma, 26*(2), 101–115. https://doi.org/10.1080/15325024.2020.1835386

Gupta, S. (Host) (2023, February 14). *How to raise kids in the digital age [Audio podcast episode]. Chasing life.* https://www.cnn.com/audio/podcasts/chasing-life/episodes/188a0639-7090-4b13-aa23-afa400d3612e

Hampton, K. N. (2019). Social media and change in psychological distress over time: The role of social causation. *Journal of Computer-Mediated Communication, 24*, 205–222.

Hoffman, B. L., Shensa, A., Escobar-Viera, C. G., Sidani, J. E., Miller, E., & Primack, B. A. (2021). "Their page is still up": Social media and coping with loss. *Journal of Loss and Trauma, 26*, 451–468.

Huang, C. (2022). A meta-analysis of the problematic social media use and mental health. *International Journal of Social Psychiatry, 68*(1), 12–33. https://doi.org/10.1177/0020764020978434

Ithnain, N., Ghazali, S. E., & Jaafar, N. (2018). Relationship between smartphone addiction with anxiety and depression among undergraduate students in Malaysia. *International Journal of Health Sciences & Research, 8*(1), 163–171.

Kircaburun, K., Demetrovics, Z., Kiraly, O., & Griffiths, M. (2020). Childhood emotional trauma and cyberbullying perpetration among emerging adults: A multiple mediation model of the role of problematic social media use and psychopathology. *International Journal of Mental Health and Addiction, 18*, 548–566.

Levaot, Y., Green, T., & Palgi, Y. (2021). Making and receiving offers of help following disaster predict posttraumatic growth but not posttraumatic stress. *Disaster Medicine Public Health Preparedness, 15*(4), 484–490.

Li, L., & Peng, W. (2019). Transitioning through social media: International students' SNS use, perceived social support, and acculturative stress. *Computers in Human Behavior, 98*, 69–79.

Louragli, I., Ahami, A., Khadmaoui, A., Aboussaleh, Y., & Lamrani, A. C. (2019). Behavioral analysis of adolescent students addicted to Facebook and its impact on performance and mental health. *ACTA Neuropsychologica, 17*(4), 427–439.

Marino, C., Canale, N., Melodia, F., Spada, M. M., & Vieno, A. (2019). The overlap between problematic smartphone use and problematic social media use: A systematic review. *Current Addiction Reports, 8,* 469–480. https://doi.org/10.1007/s40429-021-00398-0

McKay, D., & Perez, P. (2019). Citizen aid, social media and brokerage after disaster. *Third World Quarterly, 40,* 1903–1920.

McQuade, S. C., III, Colt, J. P., & Meyer, N. B. B. (2009). *Cyber bullying: Protecting kids and adults from online bullies.* Praeger.

NBC News. (2022, December). *Facebook parent META agrees to pay $725 million to settle Cambridge Analytica suit.* https://www.nbcnews.com/tech/tech-news/facebook-parent-meta-agrees-pay-725-million-settle-cambridge-analytica-rcna63081.

Pew Research Center. (2021, April 7). *Social media fact sheet.* https://www.pewresearch.org/internet/fact-sheet/social-media/

Pew Research Center. (2022a, August 10). *Teens, social media, and technology.* https://www.pewresearch.org/internet/2022/08/10/teens-social-media-and-technology-2022/

Pew Research Center. (2022b, November 16). *Connection, creativity, and drama: Teen life on social media in 2022.* https://www.pewresearch.org/internet/2022/11/16/connection-creativity-and-drama-teen-life-on-social-media-in-2022/

Prescott, J., Rathbone, A. L., & Hanley, T. (2020). Online mental health communities, self-efficacy and transition to further support. *Mental Health Review Journal, 25*(4), 329–344.

Ramazanoglu, M. (2020). The relationship between high school students' internet addiction, social media disorder, and smartphone addiction. *World Journal of Education, 10*(4), 139–148. https://doi.org/10.5430/wje.v10n4p139

Sadagheyani, H. E., & Tatari, F. (2021). Investigating the role of social media on mental health. *Mental Health and Social Inclusion, 25*(1), 41–51. https://doi.org/10.1108/MHSI-06-2020-0039

Shannon, H., Bush, K., Villenueve, P. J., Hellemans, K. G. C., & Guimond, S. (2022). Problematic social media use in adolescents and young adults: Systematic review and meta-analysis. *JMIR Mental Health, 9*(4), e33450. https://doi.org/10.2196/33450

Statista (2022, June). Number of social media users worldwide from 2017 to 2027. https://www.statista.com/statistics/278414/number-of-worldwide-social-network-users/

Stroinska, M., & Cecchetto, V. (2019). Can there be a 'safe haven' for trauma survivors in this social media dominated world? *Trames, 23*(73/68(2), 223–238.

Whiting, J. B., Pickens, J. C., Luthi Sagers, A., PettyJohn, M., & Davies, B. (2021). Trauma, social media, and #WhyIDidntReport: An analysis of twitter posts about reluctance to report sexual assault. *Journal of Marital and Family Therapy, 47,* 749–766. https://doi.org/10.1111/jmft.12470

The White House. (2022, March 1). *FACT SHEET: President Biden to announce strategy to address our national mental health crisis as part of unity agenda in his first state of the union address.* https://www.whitehouse.gov/briefing-room/statements-releases/2022/03/01/fact-sheet-president-biden-to-announce-strategy-to-address-our-national-mental-health-crisis-as-part-of-unity-agenda-in-his-first-state-of-the-union/

Zhen, L., Yuanfeixue, N., & Pham, B. (2021). College students coping with COVID-19: Stress-buffering effects of self-disclosure on social media and parental support. *Communication Research Reports, 38*(1), 23–31.

Zhong, B., Huang, Y., & Liu, Q. (2021). Mental health toll from the coronavirus: Social media usage reveals Wuhan residents' depression and secondary trauma in the COVID-19 outbreak. *Computers and Human Behavior, 114*, 1–10. https://doi.org/10.1016/j.chb.2020.106524

# Index

Printed and bound by CPI Group (UK) Ltd, Croydon, CR0 4YY

07/07/2026

14916218-0003